Food Production and Nutrition Management

CONTENT VIBES
PUBLISHERS · PRINTERS · AGGREGATORS

About the Authors

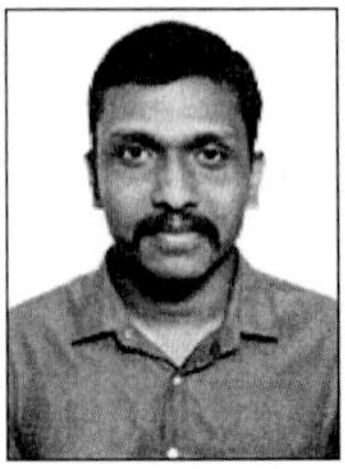

Dr. S. Prabakaran has done his B.Sc. (Agri.) from TNAU sub-campus at Trichy. He studied his M.Sc. and Ph.D. from Indian Agricultural Research Institute (IARI), New Delhi. His area of specialisation was Plant Genetic Resources. In 2015, he received ICAR-JRF 22nd rank in plant sciences and secured merit fellowship. In 2017, he secured 1st rank IARI entrance exam and secured IARI merit fellowship for Ph.D. program. He also qualified Agricultural Scientist Recruitment Board (ASRB) – National Eligibility Test (NET) in 2017. He has qualified UGC-SRF and lectureship in Environmental sciences in 2019. Currently, he is teaching agriculture optional to civil service aspirants at Chennai.

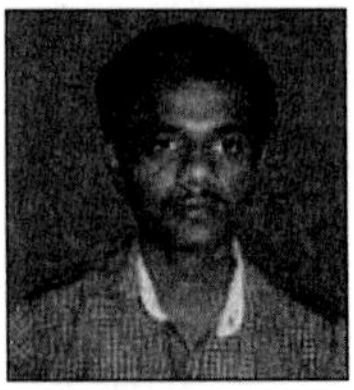

A. Krishnamoorthi I did my B.Sc. agriculture (2012-16) from VIA Agriculutre college Affiliated to TNAU and I did my Msc Agriculture in Plant geneticr esource (2108-20) from TNAU and I am written 10 book chapters 2 research article and 10 review articles I cleared my ICAR SRF Examination with Rank 4 in the Discipline of Economic Botany and Plant Genetic Resources. Now I am pursuing my Ph.D. at the ICAR-National Bureau of Plant Genetic Resources IARI Pusa Campus New Delhi.

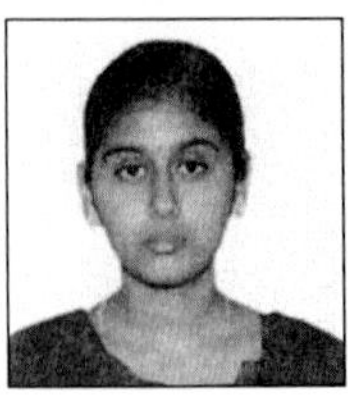

R. Sowmyapriya have studied her B.Sc. (Agri.) from TNAU sub-campus at killikulam, Tamil Nadu. She studied her M.Sc. (Biotechnology) from UAS, Bangalore. Currently, she is pursuing Ph.D. (Biotechnology) at IARI, New Delhi. She was the recipient of JNU fellowship and DBT fellowship.

Food Production and Nutrition Management

S. Prabakaran
A. Krishnamoorthi
R. Sowmyapriya

CONTENT VIBES
PUBLISHERS • PRINTERS • AGGREGATORS

CONTENT VIBES
PUBLISHERS · PRINTERS · AGGREGATORS

1168, Sector 13, Urban Estate
Karnal-132 001, Haryana
Tel: 91-84470 75807, 18440 41168
Email: contentvibesppa@gmail.com
www.contentvibes.in

Print ISBN: 978-81-97781-56-8

ebook-ISBN: 978-81-97781-53-7

Perface

In a world where the global population is projected to reach 9.7 billion by 2050, ensuring access to nutritious food is one of the most pressing challenges of our time. The double burden of malnutrition - where undernutrition coexists with overweight and obesity - affects billions of people worldwide, with far-reaching consequences for human health, economic development, and environmental sustainability.

This book, "Food Production & Nutrition Management," addresses the critical need for a comprehensive approach to food systems, one that integrates the principles of sustainable food production with the science of human nutrition. By exploring the complex relationships between agriculture, food security, and nutrition, we aim to provide a roadmap for creating healthier, more sustainable food systems.

Through a combination of theoretical foundations, real-world examples, and cutting-edge research, this book covers the entire food value chain, from crop and animal production to food processing, distribution, and consumption. We examine the impact of different production systems on nutrient quality, environmental sustainability, and human health, highlighting the need for a balanced approach that prioritizes both food security and nutrition security.

Whether you are a student, researcher, policymaker, or practitioner in the fields of agriculture, nutrition, or public health, this book invites you to join the conversation on creating a food system that nourishes both people and the planet. By exploring the intersections of food production and nutrition management, we hope to inspire new solutions, new collaborations, and a new era of food system transformation.

Ultimately, this book is a call to action - a recognition that the future of food is not just about producing more, but about producing better. Better for human health, better for the environment, and better for the well-being of all people. Join us on this journey towards a more sustainable, equitable, and nourishing food future.

Contents

1

Food Production and Consumption Trends in India

Previous Year Questions

1. *How has food production, incuding horticultural crops, changed in India during the last one decade? Write down its impact on food and nutritional security (20 marks, CSE 2023)*
2. *What is the food production and consumption pattern of India in the last fifty years? (15M, CSE 2021)*
3. *Describe food grain production and consumption trends in India (7.5M, CSE 2019)*
4. *Food production and consumption trends in India (12.5M, CSE 2015)*

Food Production Trends

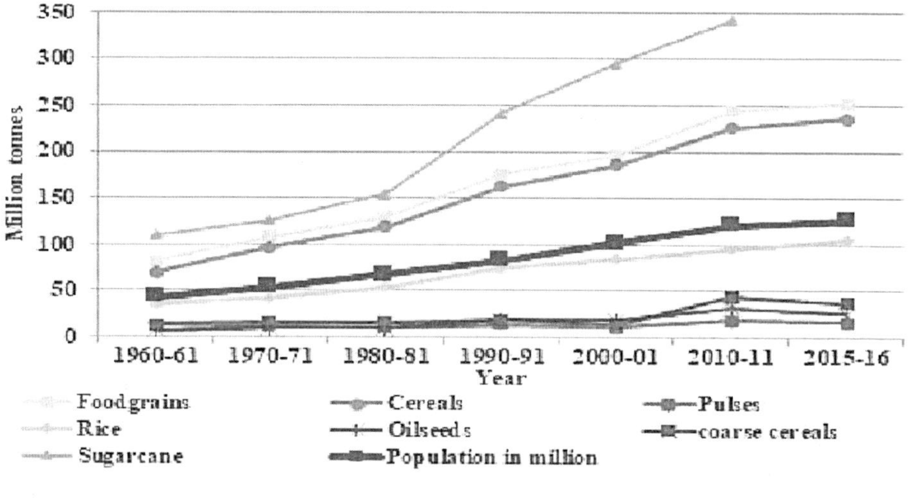

Foodgrain and Horticultural Production

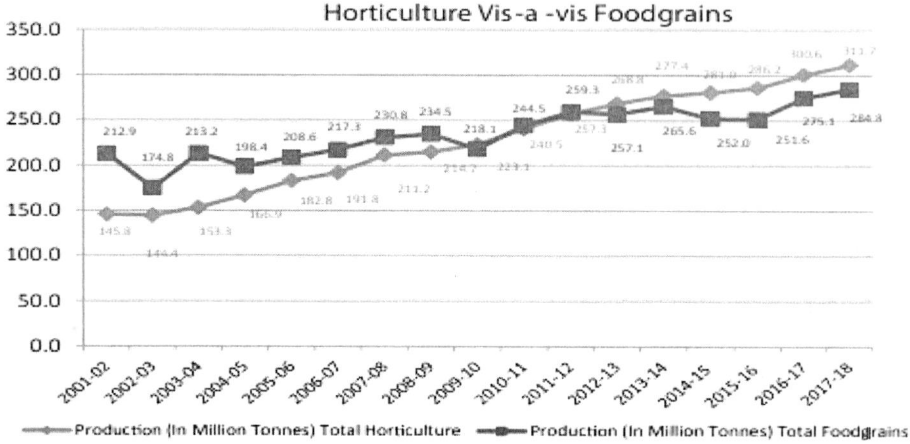

Foodgrain in 2023-330.5 MT Horticultural Production in 2023-351 MT

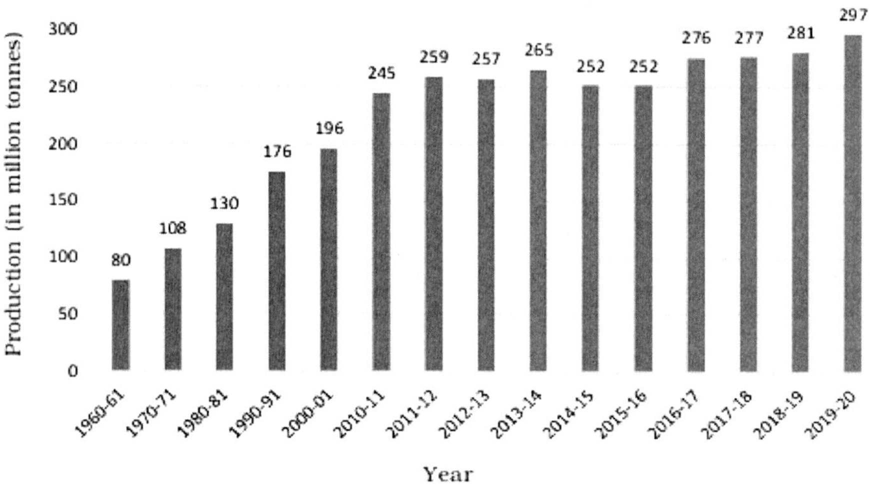

Graph 4.2: *Production of foodgrains in India (Million Tonnes)*

Source: Department of Agricultural, Cooperation and Farmers Welfare, Ministry of Agricultural and Farmers Welfare, Directorate of Economics and Statistics, 2020-21

How the Production has Increased After 1960's?

1960	11.00	34.58
1970	23.83	42.22
1980	36.31	53.63
1990	55.14	74.29
2000	69.68	84.98
2010	86.87	95.98
2017-18	102.19	116.42
2018-19	107.18	117.94
2020-21	109.24	120.32

Dr. M S Swaminathan is the "Father of the Green Revolution in India". An agricultural scientist and agronomist, he has been considered the main architect of the green revolution in India. He had a crucial role in developing the high-yielding varieties of wheat and rice, which were insect resistant and produced high-quality crops. His collaborative efforts with Norman Borlaug had made a significant impact on evading famine-like conditions in India. The World Food Prize, also known as the Nobel Prize for Food and Agriculture, was awarded for the first time in 1987 to M S Swaminathan.

Advantages of Green Revolution

i) **Food security to the nation:** Higher yield because of the utilization of HYV seeds.

ii) **Introduction of Machineries** like harvesters have made the crop cultivation quicker and simpler.

iii) **Self sufficient:** From being net food importer in the 1960s, India has emerged as a net food exporter to the world.

iv) **Benefits to the Farmers:** The introduction of the Green Revolution helped the farmers in raising their level of income. The big farmers with more than 10 hectares of land were particularly benefited by this revolution.

v) **Industrial Growth:** The Revolution brought about large scale farm mechanization which created demand for different types of machines like tractors, harvesters, threshers, combines, diesel engines, electric motors, pumping sets, etc.

Disdvantages of Green Revolution

- **Regional Disparities**: The most benifitted areas are Punjab, Haryana and western Uttar Pradesh in the north and Andhra Pradesh and Tamil Nadu in the south.

- **Replacement of agricultural labours by machines:** farm mechanization under the Green Revolution created widespread unemployment.
- **Use of synthetic chemicals:** resulted in human health hazards
- **Monoculture:** only wheat–rice cultivation
- **Depletion soil nutrients:** Repeated crop cycle in order to ensure increased crop production depleted the soil's nutrients.
- **Ground water depletion:** Irrigation pumps also sucked out the groundwater to supply the water-intensive crops, such as sugarcane and rice, thus depleting the groundwater levels.

Consumption Trends

- Indians today eat **twice as much meat, egg and fish** as they did in the early 1980s.
- **Consumption of fruits** has risen even more spectacularly - **almost three times** during the same period.
- What are being **eaten less than before are cereals** (e.g. wheat, rice) and pulses.
- The changing consumption patterns and rising exports are, in turn, driving a revolution in India's **high-value agriculture** (e.g vegetable, fruits, oil).

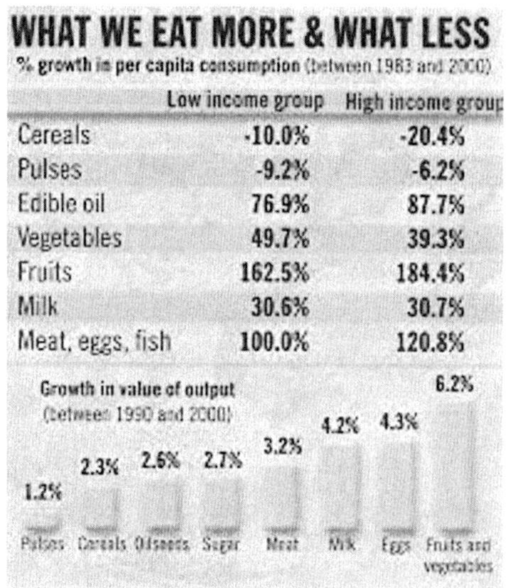

- The diet of all income groups has moved from **cereals to non-cereal foods**, whereas the focus of India's agriculture policy, institutions and public spending has always been cereals.
- **Energy intake** has increased for the poor and decreased for the rich, while **fat intake has risen** for all income groups.
- The pace of decline of **cereal consumption** in the upper-income group was faster than that of the lower-income group.
- But even among lower income groups, consumption of **high-value food** increased in the past decade.
- **Junk foods and fast food** – consumption increased in recent years.

Govt. Initiatives for Millets Consumption

- Coinciding with the **International Year of Millets 2023**, during the G 20 meetings being held in the current year, millets are being promoted on a large scale through millet melas and distribution of millet gift hampers.
- Further interaction with millet farmers are also taking place on the sidelines of the G 20 meetings to **spread the awareness about millet crops**.
- The Ministry of Food Processing Industries (MoFPI) has approved the **Production Linked Incentive Scheme** for Food Processing Industry **Millet-based products** (PLISMBP) for implementation during 2022-23 to 2026-27 with an outlay of Rs. 800 crores.

2

Food Security and Growing Population – Vision 2020

Previous Year Questions

1. ***CS 2015:*** *Discuss the impact of rapid increase in population on food and agriculture (12.5 marks)*

What is Food security?

The Food and Agricultural Organization (FAO) – "*when all people at all times have physical and economic access to sufficient, safe and nutritious food to meet their dietary needs and food preferences for an active and healthy life*".

It has Following Dimensions

- **Availability**: It means food production within the country, food imports and the stock stored in government granaries.
- **Accessibility**: It means food is within reach of every person without any discrimination.
- **Affordability:** It implies that having enough money to buy sufficient, safe and nutritious food to meet on dietary needs.

Food Security and Growing Population

- According to the United Nations, the **world population is currently at 7.8 billion.**
- This is expected to grow to 8.5 billion by 2030, 9.7 billion by 2050, and reach 11.2 billion people by the end of the century.
- Such rapid growth is associated with rising **demand for resources such as food and water.**
- From climate change to the degradation of soil health and the **rapidly decreasing availability of arable land**
- The environmental impacts of food production are **unsustainable.**

Malthusian Theory of Population

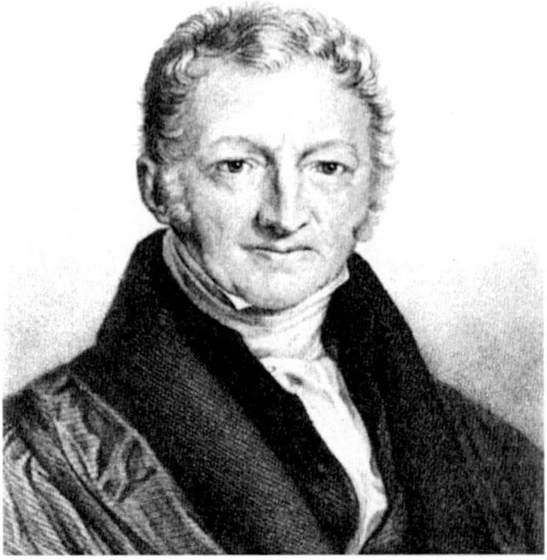

- The theory was proposed by **Thomas Robert Malthus.**
- The Malthusian Theory of Population is the theory of **exponential population and arithmetic food supply growth.**
- He believed that **a balance between population growth and food supply** can be established through preventive and positive checks.
- Food supply increases at a slower rate than the population. That is, the **food supply will be limited in a few years.**

Impact of Population Explosion on Food Security

- In India, **the population growth after independence exceeded** the agriculture growth.
- In order to maintain a balance between food and population, the annual **agriculture growth should be over 4.5%** and overall economic growth over 7%.
- At present, the annual agriculture growth is much lower being **only 3.5 percent.**
- Under the impact of rapid growth of population, the **average size of holding** has decreased to less then 1.5 hectares (1.41 ha in 1995-96; 1.08 ha in 2015-16).
- The **per capita availability of food has been decreasing** day by day.

Solutions to Population Explosion and Food Security Issues

- **Promote sustainable agriculture:** This can be achieved through measures such as promoting **agroecological practices and protecting critical ecosystems.**
- **Increase access to food:** This can be achieved through measures such as promoting economic development, investing in social safety nets and improving infrastructure for food distribution.
- **Address inequality and poverty:** This can be achieved through measures such as promoting education and employment opportunities and implementing **progressive tax policies.**

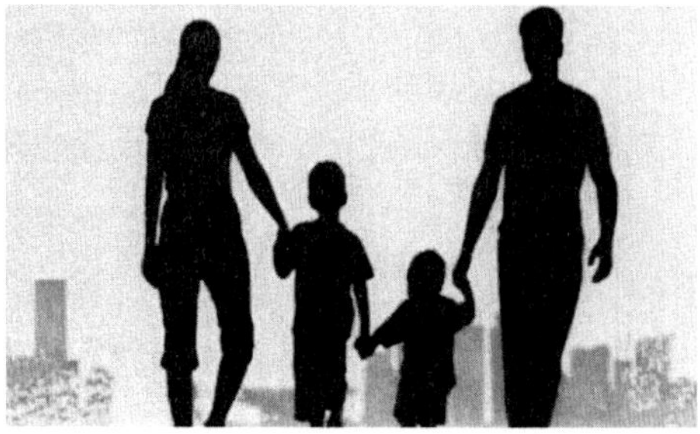

- **Population control measures:** Two child policy

- **Address climate change: This can be achieved through measures such as reducing greenhouse gas emissions, promoting climate-resilient agriculture, and investing in renewable energy.**

Strategy under Vision -2020

Research Relevance

- Research planning and prioritization as a **bottom-up initiative**
- Promote **participatory approach** for conducting research

Equity

- Bring in **decentralization** of agricultural research management
- **Removal of regional imbalance** for institutional infrastructure and human

Diversified Agriculture

- **Diversify agriculture** with focus on horticulture, livestock, fisheries and agroforestry
- Special attention to **post-production technology,** value-addition, agri-business management and trade

Efficiency

- Develop a research system with resources that provide **sufficient social benefits per unit of research inputs** and add value for investment
- Achieve **small farm mechanization and precision farming**
- Ensure technological **empowerment of women** in agriculture resources

Environmental Sustainability

- System-based **interdisciplinary research** thrust
- Concern for **conservation and effective use** of life-support systems, e.g. soil, water, flora, fauna and the atmosphere
- **Organic recycling** and waste and byproduct utilization
- Addressing **global climate change.**

Resource

- **Training in frontier sciences, technologies** and agricultural research management
- Enhancement in **vocational skills**
- Thrust on **manpower planning**

Partnership

- **Complimentarity in research efforts** among institutions and agencies at the national and international levels
- **Public-private** sector linkages
- Effective role of stakeholders (**Farmers' Associations, NGOs, Public and private sectors** etc.)

Infrastructure

- Develop efficient infrastructure for **agricultural research, education and extension education**

3

Reason for Grain Surplus

Previous Year Questions

1. *Discuss the reasons for food grain surplus (7.5 marks, CSE 2019)*
2. *What are the reasons for good grain surplus in India? Write the steps taken by the government to save the food grains. (12.5M, CSE 2015)*

Reason for Grain Surplus

Green Revolution

- Introduction of **high yielding varieties of Rice and Wheat**
- Green Revolution was made possible through the use of
- Improved irrigation, Fertilisers, Insecticides, Weedicides
- Agriculture finance at low interest rate.

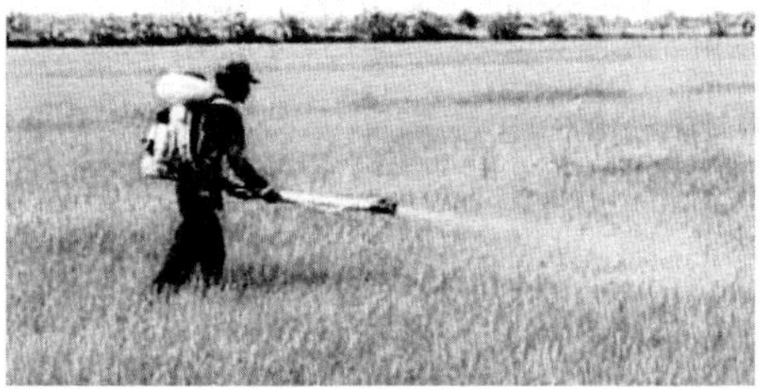

High Yielding Varieties

- These seeds are more productive. Consequent to the use of HYV seeds, the production of food grains in **1967-68 increased by 25%**

Agricultural Machineries

- Widespread introduction and use of equipment such **as tractors, combine harvesters, and sprayers.**
- The use of **machines reduced production costs** and was faster than manual labor.
- For large-scale farms, this **increased their efficiency** and thereby created economies of scale.

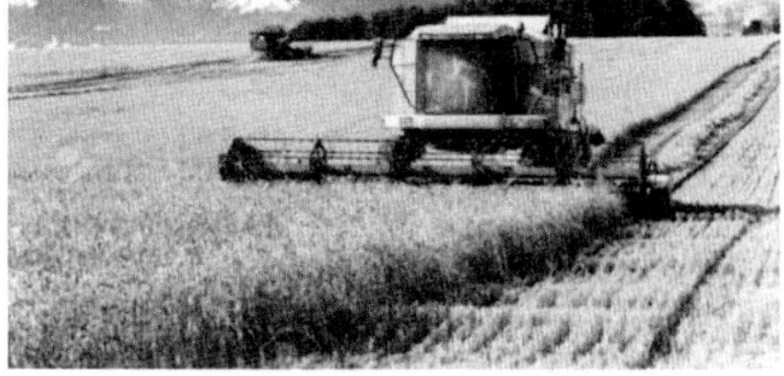

Reason for Grain Surplus

Minimum Support Price

- The MSP is the rate at which the **government purchases crops from farmers**, and is based on a calculation of at least one-and-a-half times the cost of production incurred by the farmers.
- **Skewed MSP dominated system of rice and wheat** leads to overproduction of these crops and discourages farmers to grow other crops and horticulture products.

FCI Procurement

- As against the official announcement of MSP for 23 crops, **only two, rice and wheat, are procured** as these are distributed in NFSA (National Food Security Act).

Extension Programmes

- IAAP, IADP, HYV etc led to **transfer of technology of major cereal crops** like Rice and wheat.

Double-Cropping System

- **Dams were created,** as well as other rudimentary irrigation systems.
- Instead of having only one agricultural season every year, **it was decided to have two.**
- Because there is just one rainy season every year, the one-season-per-year practise was adopted.
- The second phase's water came from massive irrigation installations.

Reason for Grain Surplus

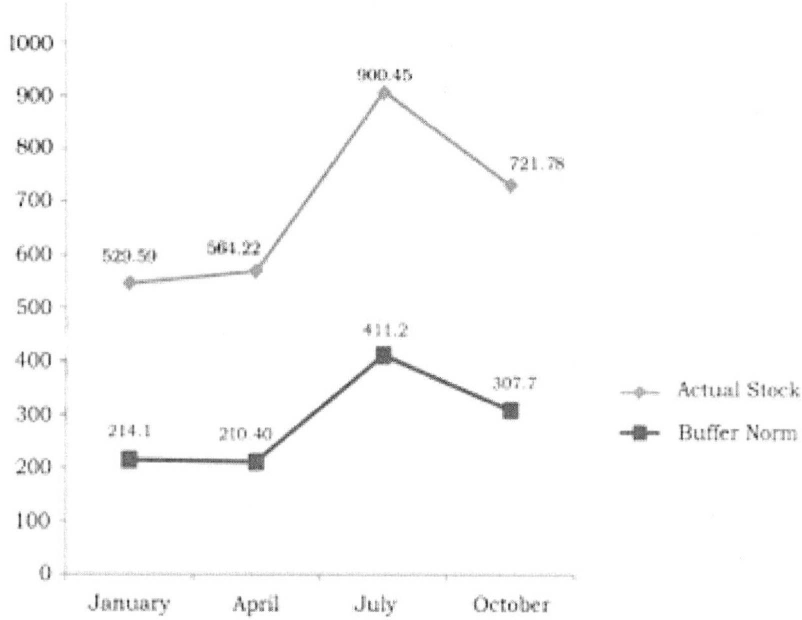

Graph 4.2: *Central foodgrains (Wheat + Rice) Stock and Minimum Buffer Norm (Million Tonnes)*

Source: Food Corporation and India (dfpd.gov.in/foodgrain-stocking). 2020-21

Steps Taken by Govt. to Save Food Grains

- All godowns are to be **constructed as per specifications.**
- Foodgrains are to be stored by adopting proper **scientific code of storage practices.**
- Adequate **dunnage materials** such as wooden crates, bamboo mats, polythene sheets are to be used to check migration of moisture from the floor to the foodgrains.
- Fumigation covers, nylon ropes, nets and **insecticides for control of stored grain insect pests** are to be provided in all the godowns.
- Prophylactic (spraying of insecticides) and **curative treatments (fumigation)** are to be carried out regularly and timely in godowns for the control of stored grain insect pests.
- **Effective rat control measures**, both in covered godowns as well as in CAP storage are to be used.
- Steel silos vs Cover and plinth shown below

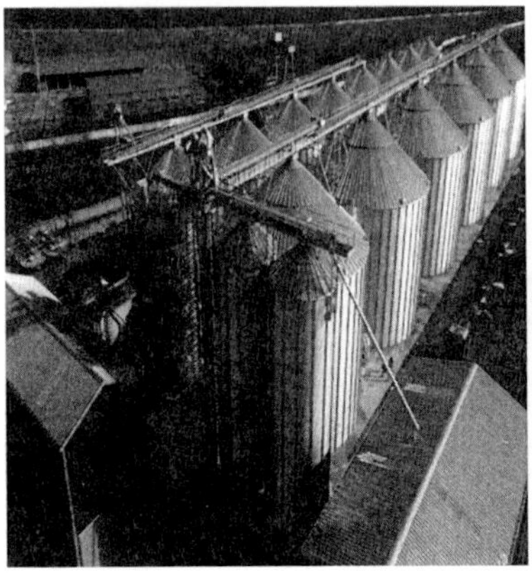

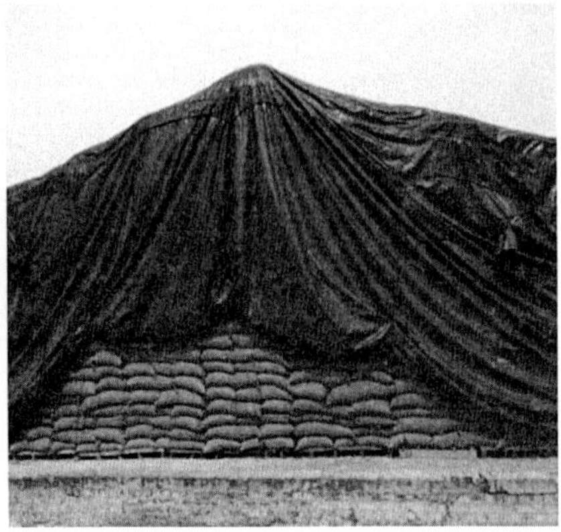

- Foodgrains in **'Cover and Plinth' (CAP) storage** are to be stored on elevated plinths and wooden crates are to be used as dunnage material.
- Stacks are to be properly covered with specifically fabricated low-density black **polythene water -proof covers** and tied with nylon ropes/ nets.
- **Regular periodic inspections** of the stocks/godowns are to be undertaken by qualified and trained staff and all senior officers.
- The principle of **"First in First Out" (FIFO)** is to be followed to the extent possible so as to avoid longer storage of foodgrains in godowns.
- Only **covered rail wagons are to be used** for movement of foodgrains so as to avoid damage during transit.

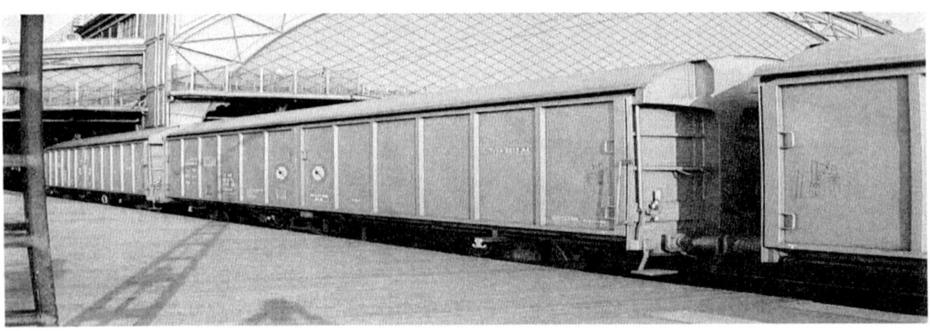

4

National and International Food Policies

Previous Year Questions

1. *Write down the various programmes run by state & central govts for ensuring food security in our country. Briefly discuss the strategies for sustainable agricultural production (20M, CSE 2023)*
2. *How will national food policy help in sustainable food security? (CSE 2020, 10 marks)*
3. *Discuss the national initiatives for food and nutrition security. (8M, IFoS-2019)*
4. *What are the special schemes for providing food grains to underprivileged, destitutes and malnourished populations (CSE 2016, 12.5 marks)*
5. *National and international food policies. (10M, IFoS-2016)*

National Food Policies / Schemes /Act / Programmes

- The Indian Constitution **does not have any explicit provision** regarding right to food.
- However, the fundamental right to life enshrined in **Article 21** of the Constitution may be interpreted to include right to live with human dignity, which may include the **right to food and other basic necessities.**

1. National Food Security Act, 2013

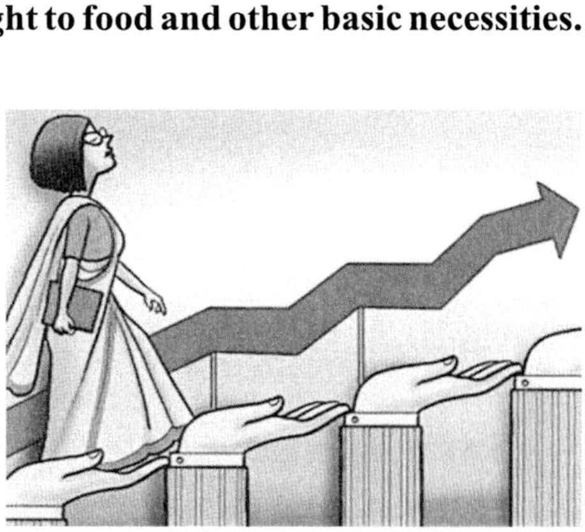

- Paradigm shift in the approach to food security from **welfare to rights based approach.**
- The Act legally entitles upto **75% of the rural population & 50% of the urban population** to receive subsidized foodgrains under Targeted Public Distribution System.

- About **two thirds of the population** therefore is covered under the Act to receive highly subsidized foodgrains.
- As a step towards **women empowerment**, the eldest woman of the household of age 18 years or above is mandated to be the head of the household for the purpose of issuing of ration cards under the Act.

Coverage

- The Act is being implemented in all the States/UTs, and on an all India basis, out of **maximum coverage of 81.34 crore persons**, have been covered under NFSA at present for receiving highly subsidized foodgrains.
- Food security allowances rules, 2015

Life Cycle Approach

- Special provisions have been made for **pregnant women and lactating mothers and children** in the age group of 6 months to 14 years.
- The act entitled them to receive nutritious meal free of cost through a widespread network of Integrated Child Development Services (ICDS) centres, called **Anganwadi Centres under ICDS scheme** and also through schools under Mid-Day Meal (MDM) scheme.
- Higher nutritional norms have been prescribed for **malnourished children upto 6 years of age.**
- **Pregnant women and lactating mothers are further entitled to receive cash maternity benefit of not less than Rs. 6,000 to partly compensate for the wage loss during the period of pregnancy and also to supplement nutrition. i) Priority House Hold (PHH)**
- Entitled to receive **5 kg of food-grains per person per month** at subsidized prices from the ration shops not exceeding
- ₹ 3 (Three) per kg of rice,
- ₹ 2 (Two) per kg of wheat and
- ₹ 1 (One) per kg for coarse grains for a period fixed by the Central Government.

Inclusion Criteria

- Household without shelter.
- Household with destitute who is living on alms.
- All households of primitive tribal groups.
- Household having a widow pension holder, if not otherwise ineligible as

per the nine exclusion criteria.

- A person with disabilities of 40% or more.
- Any transgender person.

Exclusion Criteria

- Any household that has a pucca roof with a minimum of three rooms with pucca walls.
- Households paying income tax.
- Households comprising pensioners or a member who earns more than Rs.10,000 on a monthly basis in a rural area and Rs.15,000 in an urban area.
- Households with a regular employee – gazetted or non-gazetted of State Government, Central Government, Public Sector Undertakings, Government aided local and autonomous bodies.
- Households with a domestic electric connection with a load of 2 KW or more; consumes about 300 units of energy (KWH) on a monthly basis.
- Households that have enterprises registered with the government for services and manufacturing.
- Any household that has a motorized vehicle, a four-wheeler, a heavy vehicle, a trawler, two or more motorboats.
- Households with mechanised agricultural equipment such as tractors, and harvesters.

ii) Antyodaya Anna Yojana Ration Card

- It is estimated that 5**% of people unable to get two square meals a day** on a sustained basis throughout the year.
- Their purchase is so low that they are not in a position to buy food grains round the year even at BPL rates
- **5 crores of people or 1 crore families** which constitutes the target group of Antyodya Anna Yojana.
- To serve the **poorest of the poor** in rural and urban areas.

Benefits

- 35 kg of food grain per household per month.
- **Wheat and rice** are being issued at the scale of **15 kg and 20 kg per family per month** at the rate of Rs. 2 and Rs. 3 per kg respectively.

Criteria for Antyodaya Anna Yojana Ration Card

- Landless agriculture labourers
- Marginal farmers
- Rural artisans/craftsmen such as potters, tanners, weavers, blacksmiths, carpenters, slum dwellers, and persons earning their livelihood on daily basis in the informal sector like porters, coolies, rickshaw pullers, hand cart pullers, fruit and flower sellers, snake charmers, rag pickers, cobblers, destitute and other similar categories in both rural and urban areas.
- Households headed by widows or terminally ill persons / disabled persons / persons aged 60 years or more with no assured means of subsistence or societal support.
- Widows or terminally ill persons or disabled persons or persons aged 60 years or more or single women or single men with no family or societal support or assured means of subsistence.
- All primitive tribal households.

iii) Annapurna Yojna Ration Card

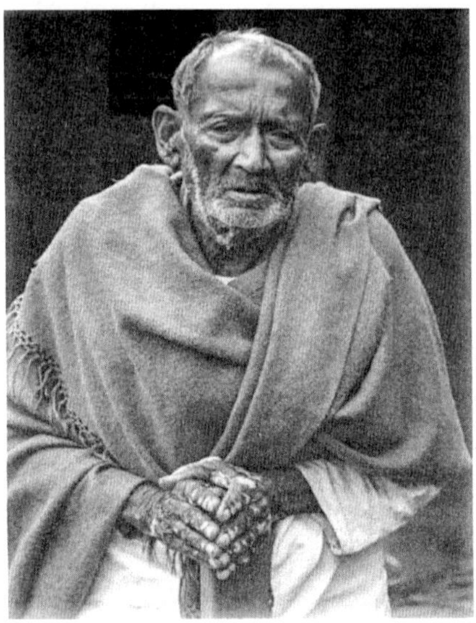

- Annapurna Scheme was launched in the year 2000 with effect from 1st April by the **Ministry of Rural Development.**
- It is a Central Sector Scheme. It is one of the sub-scheme of the National Assistance Program.
- Annapurna Yojna (AY) Ration Card is a special type of ration card issued **only to the elderly poor people above 65 years.**
- They are entitled for **10kgs of food grain** on the monthly basis from the government side.
- This food assistance is provided to those senior citizens who are eligible but **not included in the National Old Age Pension Scheme.**

iv) Non-Priority Categories (NPHH)

- The house holds remaining after selecting priority list will be moved to Non-Priority category.
- Non Priority House Holds (NPHH) are ineligible to get subsidised food grains under NFSA system.
- According to NFSA, 25% of the rural population and 50% of urban population will be out from receiving subsidized food-grains under Targeted Public Distribution System (TPDS).
- They will get ration cards but no subsidized food grains as priority ration cards (PHH) get.

2. Mid-day meal scheme / PM - POSHAN

About: It is the largest school feeding programme of its kind in the world, covering students enrolled in government schools from Classes 1 to 8.

Basic objective: to enhance enrolment in schools.

Nodal Ministry: Ministry of Education.

Background

- The programme was first introduced in 1925 for disadvantaged children in Madras Municipal Corporation.
- The union government launched as a centrally sponsored scheme on a pilot basis in 1995 for children in Classes 1 to 5.
- By October 2007, MDMS had been scaled up to Class 8.

Scale of Coverage: The scheme covers 11.80 crore children across Classes 1 to 8 (age group 6 to 14).

Legal Entitlement: It is not just a scheme, but a legal entitlement of all school-going children in primary and upper primary classes, through the National Food Security Act (NFSA), 2013.

Mid-day Meal Scheme Norms

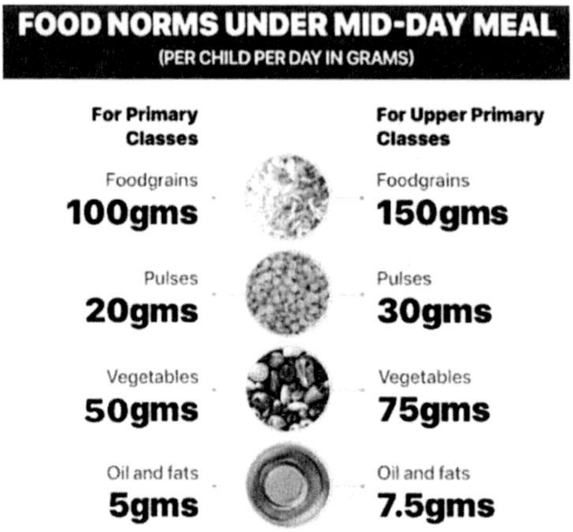

3. Integrated Child Development Scheme

Anganwadi Services Scheme

- It is a unique programme for **early childhood care and development.**
- The beneficiaries under the Scheme are **children in the age group of 0-6 years, pregnant women and lactating mothers.**
- It provides a package of six services namely **supplementary nutrition, pre-school non-formal education, nutrition & health education, immunisation, health check-up and referral services.**
- Supplementary Nutrition includes **Take Home Ration (THR), Hot Cooked Meal and morning snacks** holds importance for many vulnerable households as it impacts the nutritional outcome of the children.

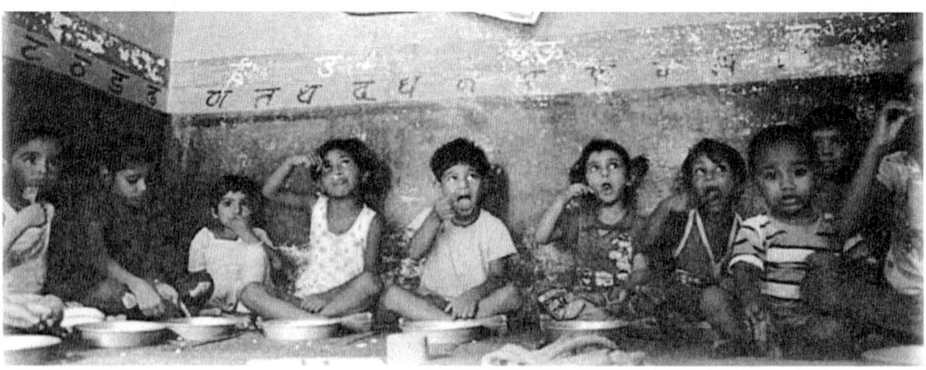

4. Pradhan Mantri Garib Kalyan Anna Yojana (PMGKAY)

- To help the poor fight the **battle against Covid-19.**
- The scheme aimed at providing each person who is covered under the National Food Security Act 2013 with an **additional 5 kg grains (wheat or rice) for free**, in addition to the 5 kg of subsidised foodgrain already provided through the Public Distribution System (PDS).
- It was initially announced for a three-month period (April, May and June 2020), covering 80 crore cardholders.
- Later it was extended **till September 2022** Merger of PMGKAY and NFSA:
- In January 2023, the PMGKAY was integrated with the NFSA, resulting in **the provision of all rations for AAY and PHH families at no cost.**
- This merger eliminated the extra provisions that were introduced during the Covid-19 pandemic by incorporating the **free component of the PMGKAY into the NFSA**

International Initiatives

1. Food and Agricultural Organization (FAO)

- Established as a specialized agency of the United Nations in 1945.
- One of FAO's strategic objectives is to help **eliminate hunger, food insecurity, and malnutrition.**

2. World Food Programme (WFP)

- Founded in 1963, WFP is the lead UN agency that responds to food emergencies and has **programmes to combat hunger worldwide.**

3. International Fund for Agricultural Development (IFAD)

- Founded in 1977, IFAD focuses on rural poverty reduction, working with poor rural populations in developing countries to **eliminate poverty, hunger, and malnutrition.**
- It is a specialized agency of the United Nations and was one of the major outcomes of the **1974 World Food Conference.**

4. World Bank

- Founded in 1944, the World Bank is actively involved in **funding food projects and programmes**.

5. High-Level Task Force (HLTF) on Global Food & Nutrition Security

- It aims to promote a comprehensive and unified response of the international community to the challenge of **achieving global food and nutrition security.**
- It was established by the **UN Secretary-General Ban Ki-moon** in 2008.

6. Zero Hunger Challenge in 2012

During the Rio+20 World Conference on Sustainable Development. The Zero Hunger Challenge was launched to inspire a **global movement towards a world free from hunger** within a generation. It calls for:

- Zero stunted children under the age of two
- 100% access to adequate food all year round
- 100% increase in smallholder productivity and income
- Zero loss or waste of food

5

Production, Procurement, Distribution Constraints; Processing Constraints

Previous Year Questions

1. *Write down the constraints of fruit processing industry in India (10M, CSE 2023)*
2. *Enlist & Explain the issues & challenges in the growth of food processing industry in India (10M, CSE 2022)*
3. *Give a detailed account of constraints in sustaining the food-grain production in India. (10M, IFoS 2020)*
4. *What are the major constraints of food production in India (10 mark, CSE 2020)*
5. *Describe the food production constraints in Indian agricultural system. (15M, IFoS-2018)*
6. *Indicate the major constraints in food procurement and distribution. (10M, CSE 2017)*
7. *Discuss the procurement and processing constraints of food grain. (15M, IFoS-2017)*

Production Constraints

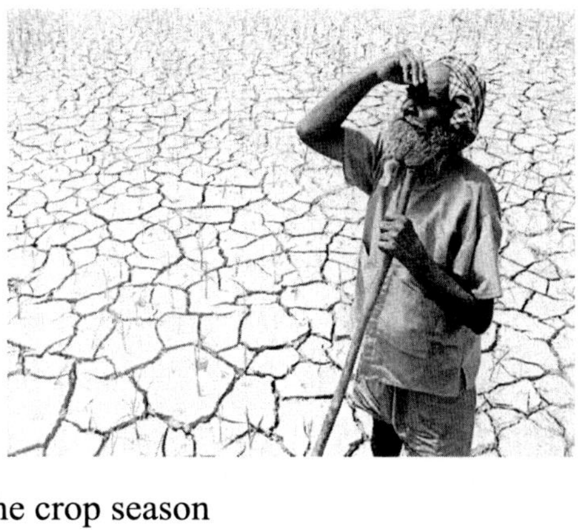

- Lack of awareness about the latest technical knowledge of the crop
- Lack of recommended package of practices of the major food grains at the ground level
- limitation of resources i.e. seeds, water , equipment etc.
- Lack of sufficient soil testing facilities in area
- Unavailability of labour during the crop season

- Insufficient fund to purchase different inputs for crop cultivation.
- Delays in receiving Funds received for crop production from financial institution.
- Problem to get machines on hire basis for crop production
- Monsoon failure

Lack of Access to Credit & Finance

- Small and marginal farmers often face **difficulties in accessing credit and financial services.**
- Limited availability of affordable credit **restricts their ability to invest in modern farming** equipment and quality seeds and fertilizers, hampering their productivity.

Small landholdings

- Average farmers are small landholders, leading to **fragmented and uneconomical farming practices.**

Outdated Farming Practices

- A significant portion of Indian farmers still rely on **traditional and outdated farming methods.**
- **Lack of awareness about modern techniques** and resistance to change hinder the adoption of advanced farming practices.

Water Scarcity & Irrigation

- India's agriculture is **heavily dependent on monsoon rain**, making it vulnerable to droughts and inconsistent rainfall patterns.
- **Access to irrigation facilities** and water management are crucial challenges, particularly in regions with limited water resources.

Soil Degradation & Land Erosion

- Improper land use practices, **excessive use of chemical fertilizers and pesticides** and inadequate soil conservation measures contribute to soil degradation and erosion.
- This leads to reduced soil fertility
- Increased vulnerability to pests and diseases,
- Reduced agricultural productivity.

Market Volatility & Price Fluctuations

- Farmers in India often **face price volatility** due to lack of effective market linkages, intermediaries and price information.

- This leaves them vulnerable to **price exploitation** and uncertain returns on their investments.

Climate Change & Natural Disasters

- Increasingly **unpredictable weather patterns, climate change and occurrences of natural disasters**—such as floods, cyclones and droughts—pose significant challenges to the country's agriculture industry.
- These events can lead to **crop losses, livestock** mortality and increased vulnerability for farmers.

Procurement Constraints (Based on Standing Committee Report)

Refusing Procurement at Centres

- The Committee noted that lower staff posted at procurement centres sometimes **refuse to procure on non-bonafide technical reasons**, such as moisture content in the produce.

Construction of Godowns

- The Committee observed that **FCI could not achieve the targets for construction** of godowns in 2020-21.
- Recommended construction of mini godowns in different parts of the states.

Damaged Foodgrains

- The Committee noted a very high value of **damaged foodgrains during 2017-20 (Rs 12.6 crore).**
- It noted that damaged foodgrains accrued mainly due to **pest attacks, exposure to rain, floods, leakages in godowns, procurement of poor quality stocks, and negligence of officials.**

  Very slow movement of foodgrains to distribution centres, which leads to huge **piling of foodgrains and rotting.**

Transit losses

- The Committee noted that despite various initiatives of the Department to reduce storage and transit losses of foodgrains, **transit losses are still very high (Rs 281 crore during April-October 2020).**

Decentralised Procurement

- Under the Decentralised Procurement Scheme (introduced in 1997-98), the state governments utilise the **foodgrains procured locally from within the state** for distribution under various schemes.

- The Committee observed that even after 23 years of the inception of the scheme, it has been **undertaken by only 8 states** in case of wheat, and 15 states in case of rice.

Distribution Constraints

- **'Ghost' card holders:** The Gram Panchayats and the Gram Sabhas are given responsibility of identification, but in states where these bodies are not functional, **PDS dealers are seen performing the task and benefitting from it.**

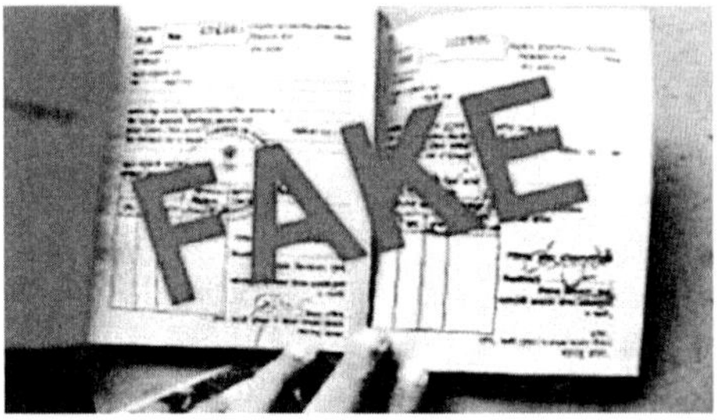

Leakages and Diversion

- **More than half (54%) of the grain** taken off for TPDS disappeared before they reached buyers in the fair price shop.
- NSSO 68th round reports that **diversion of grains from PDS amounts to 46.7%** in 2011-12. Diversion of Food grains by Fair Price Shops holder and mediator.
  - **Irregular arrival of grains in fair price shop:** Because of lack of awareness among poor households about the **exact arrival of grains** creates the problem of physical & economic access.

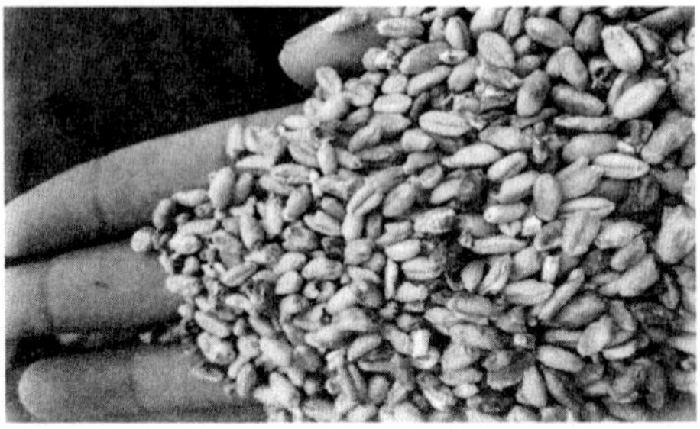

  - **Quality of food items:** The quality of food items provided through the PDS system is **often poor,** leading to health-related issues.
  - Identification of poor by the states is not fool proof. A **large number of poor and needy persons are left out** and a lot of fake cards are also issued.
  - People **do not get the permitted amount of food grains** from the Fair price shop.
  - Many times, good quality food grains are **replaced with poor quality** cheap food grains.
  - Public distribution system includes only few food grains such as wheat and rice, it **does not fulfil the requirement of complete nutrition.**

- **Uneven distribution of Food generations, procurement and distribution:** North eastern states are very far from Punjab and Haryana, from where wheat is procured.
- To transport food grains **from Punjab to far flung areas in North east** will entail cost and time both.

Processing Constraints

Poor laboratories Quality Standards

- The large number of entities participating in the food value chain, particularly in the big unorganized portion, makes **enforcing quality and safety standards challenging.**
- As a result, procedures like **milk adulteration and the use of carbide** for fruit ripening have become increasingly common.

Poor marketability of Processed Products

- An **insufficient link** between production and processing;
- **Seasonality** of operations and poor capacity utilization;

Low Access to Credit and Subsidized Financing

- Despite the introduction of the Food Processing Fund a few years ago, the industry has been suffering from a **lack of resources**.
- Even if a foreign investment has increased recently, it still falls short of the industry's needs.

Low Value-Added in Processing

- A large unorganized segment and widespread use of **primitive processing.**
- This results in **lower value-addition** at the processing stage, especially from a nutritional point of view.

Logistics Issues

- Logistics in India still face challenges related to **quality and connectivity:**
- Indian NH account for only 2% of the total road network but carry 40% of all cargo.

Other Issues

- **Lack of applied research, Taxation issues, obsolete technologies** etc. persist in the sector.

Large Informalisation

- More than 50% of the industries in the food processing sector is concentrated in **informal sector and are small scale industries.**
- They **cannot achieve economy of scale** & avail the benefits from the formal financial sector.

Govt. Schemes Related to Food Processing

Pradhan Mantri Kisan SAMPADA Yojana

- In 2016, MoFPI introduced an umbrella **Scheme for Agro-Marine Processing and Development of Agro-Processing Clusters (SAMPADA),** which was proposed to be implemented with an allocation of ₹6,000 crores for the period of 2016-20.
- In 2017, SAMPADA was renamed as the **Pradhan Mantri Kisan Sampada Yojana (PMKSY).**
- It is a Central Sector Scheme.

Implementation of Kisan SAMPADA Yojana

- The Ministry of Food Processing Industries (MOFPI) has approved the establishment of **42 Mega Food Parks, 236 Integrated Cold Chains** with a view to creating a modern infrastructure for food processing along the value chain from the farm to the market.

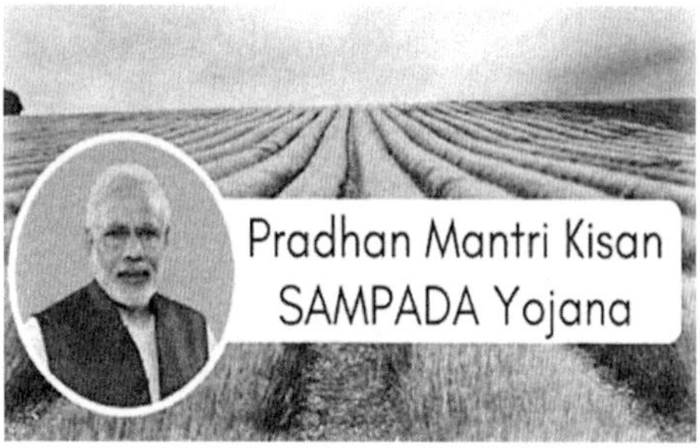

- Steps are being taken to boost the food processing sector in order to fulfill the objectives of bringing down **post-harvest wastages and losses preferably to zero levels.**
- The scheme intends to **identify agro clusters and grant them subsidies** so that the transfer of food products from the producing centres to the market becomes seamless.
- SAMPADA aims at the entire linkage and plugging gaps in the supply chain, **modernization/ expansion of existing food processing units,** creation of processing and preservation capacities, etc.
- The scheme will benefit the farmers by increasing their income, generate employment opportunities, **stimulate the export of processed food** and reduce food wastage.

6

Availability of Food Grains, Per Capita Expenditure on Food

Previous Year Questions

1. *No questions were asked in past 10 years*

Availability of Foodgrains

- **Net availability of foodgrains** = Gross Production (-) seed, feed & wastage, (-) exports imports (+/-) change in stocks.
- **Per capita availability of foodgrains (kg/yr)**

$$= \frac{\text{The net availability of foodgrains}}{\text{Population estimates for a particular year}}$$

- **Net availability of foodgrains in terms of grams/days**

$$= \frac{\text{Per capita availability of foodgrains (kg / yr)}}{\text{365 day}} * 1000$$

- Annual availability of food grains in India for fiscal year 2021 -22 amounted to about **187 Kilograms per capita.**
- There has been a **consistent increase in the availability of food grains** annually since 2015.

(000 Tonnes Unless Otherwise Stated)							(As on 23.1 1.2022)	
Year	Population in thousand persons	Production		Net Imports	Change in Stocks	Net availability	Per Capita Net Availability	
		Cross	Net				Kg. per year	Grams per day
Rice								
2018-19	1338995	116478	107626	-12056	4521	91049	68	186.3
2019-20	1353378	118870	109836	-9505	2845	97485	72	197.3
2020-21	1367173	124370	114918	-17775	-3121	100264	73.3	200.9
2021-22	1379750	130291	120389	-21222	3204	95963	69.6	190.5
Wheat								
2018-19	1338995	103596	91061	-224	3761	87076	65	178.2
2019-20	1353378	107860	94809	-218	7708	86883	64.2	175.9
2020-21	1367173	109590	96330	-2155	2604	91571	67	183.5
2021-22	1379750	106845	93917	-7244	-8314	94987	68.8	188.6
Foodgrains								
2018-19	1338995	285209	255680	-11052	8965	235663	176	482.2
2019-20	1353378	297500	266567	-6885	11814	247867	183,1	501.8
2020-21	1367173	310740	278430	-20681	2400	255348	186.8	511.7
2021-22	1379750	315720	283071	-30003	-6090	259158	187.8	514.6

Per Capita Expenditure on Food

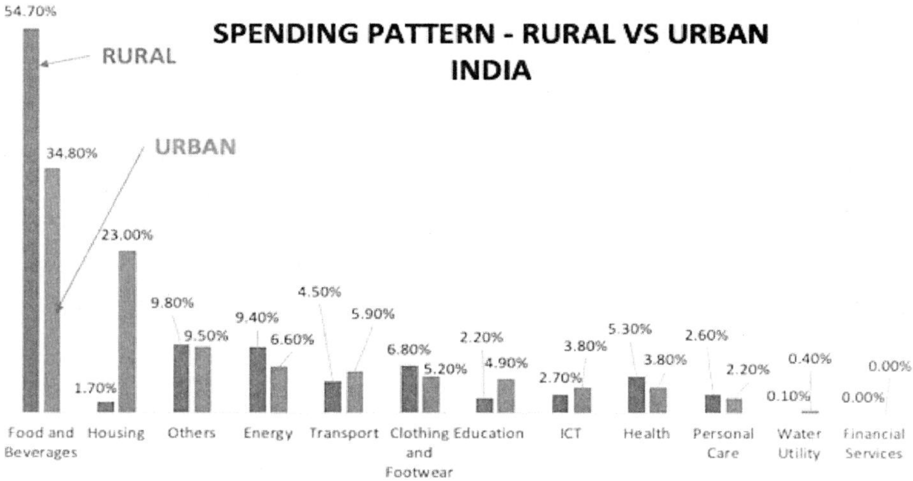

Per Capita Expenditure on Food

Rural India

- Per Capita Consumption of Rural India is Rs.12,662.89 per year.
- On an average, a household in India has 4.922 people people.
- Means, a rural Indian family spends about Rs.62,326.74 per year (=12662.89×4.922).
- Out of Rs.62,326 **food and beverages consume 54.7%.**
- Rural India also spend more (compared to Urban) on **clothing & footwear, health, personal care.**

Urban India

- Per Capita Consumption of Urban India is Rs.28,956.05 per year.
- Considering 4.922 people per household, an urban Indian family spends about Rs.1,42,521.67 per year (=28956.89×4.922).
- Out of Rs.1,42,521 **food and beverages consume 34.8%, and housing consumes 23%.**
- Urban India also spends more on **transport, education and communication.**

7

Trends in Poverty, Public Distribution System and Below Poverty Line Population Targeted Public Distribution System (PDS), Policy Implementation in Context to Globalization

Previous Year Questions

1. *Discuss the strengths and weaknesses of Public Food Distribution system in India. (8M, IFoS-2022)*
2. *Describe the vicious cycle of poverty and enlist the existing policy instruments for combating malnutrition. (20M, CSE 2022)*
3. *Enlist and explain the efforts of the GOI in streamlining the current levels of poverty (10 marks, CS 2022)*
4. *Enlist and explain the salient features of Public Distribution System as per the provisions of the National Food Security Act, 2013. (10M, CSE 2022)*
5. *Discuss the strengths and weaknesses of public food-grain distribution system in India. (8M, IFoS 2020)*
6. *What is Public Distribution System (PDS) and what are its objectives? How does targeted public distribution system overcome problem with PDS? (15M, CSE 2020)*
7. *Discuss the strength & weakness of public distribution system in the country. (10M, 150W, CSE 2016)*
8. *What do you mean by Targeted Public Distribution System (TPDS)? Who are specially focussed group covered under this programme? (10M, 150W, CSE 2015)*
9. *GS– III question 2022: What are the major challenges of Public Distribution Sytem in India? How can it be made effective & transparent? (150 words)*

What is poverty?

- Poverty is said to exist "**when people lack the means to satisfy their basic needs**".

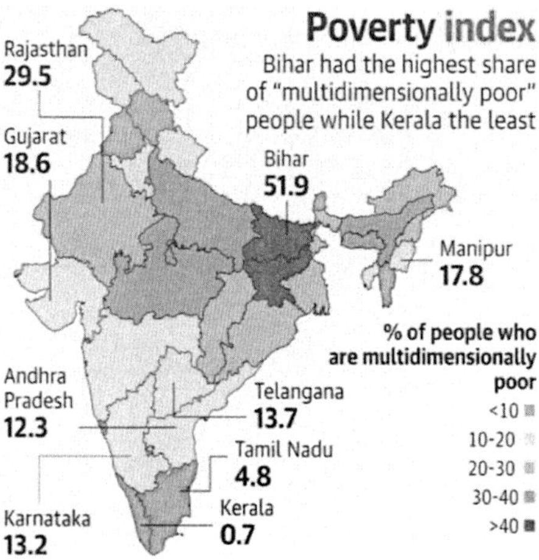

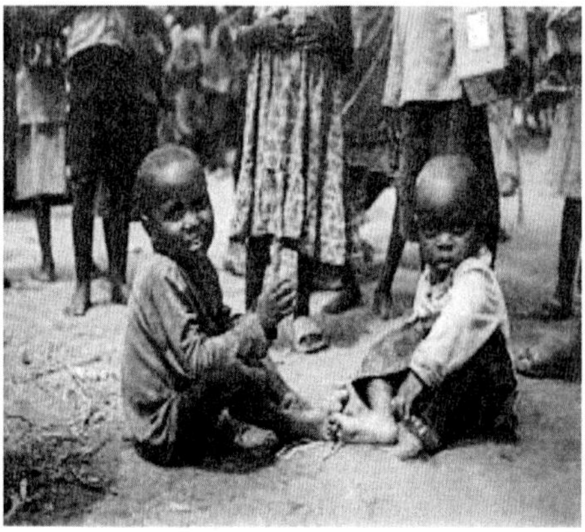

Absolute and Relative poverty

Absolute Poverty	Relative Poverty
Concept	
Absolute poverty is the traditionally accepted concept of poverty.	The concept of relative poverty has been put forward by Prof. Peter Townsend.
Definition	
"Lack of income to satisfy basic requirements of life ie food, clothing and shelter essential for survival".	"A situation where people are deprived of their customary living standards of the society in which they live".
Cause	
Lack of income, low PCI. low PCC. etc.	Differences in income.
Nature	
Absolute poverty is not universal in nature, it may or may not exist in a country.	Relative poverty is universal in nature, it exists in all country
Measure	
Increase in income, control of population, increase in employment etc will reduce absolute poverty.	Reduction in the gap between rich and poor. a more equal distribution of income will reduce relative poverty.
With Reference To Poverty Line	
Absolutely poor people live below the poverty line.	Relatively poor people may live on. above or below the poverty line

Results In	
A large extent of absolute poverty [When more than 50% of population is absolutely poor], results in "MASS POVERTY".	A large extent of relative poverty results in "INEQUATY".
Other Points	
Absolute poverty can be completely eradicated.	Relative poverty can never be completely eradicated.

Poverty estimates by different committees

Year	Lakdwala Committee Estimates			Tendulker Committee Estimates			Rangarajan Committee Estimates		
	Rural	Urban	Total	Rural	Urban	Total	Rural	Urban	Total
1993-94	37.3	32.4	36.0	50.1	31.8	45.3	-	-	-
2004-05	28.3	25.7	27.5	41.8	25.7	37.2	-	-	-
2009-10	-	-	-	33.8	20.9	29.8	39.6	35.1	38.2
2011-12	-	-	-	25.7	13.7	21.9	30.9	26.4	29.5

Pre- Independence Estimation of Poverty

- Dadabhai Naoroji took concrete steps in identifying the poor people in India. He had formulated a plan that ranged from Rs 16 to Rs 35 per capita per year based on 1867-68 prices of subsistence diet.
- National Planning Committee (1938) devised a poverty line ranging from Rs 15 to Rs 20 per capita per month. It was based on a minimum standard of living where nutritional requirements are very important.
- Bombay Plan (1944) suggested a poverty line of Rs 75 per capita per year.

Post- Independence Estimation of Poverty

1. VN Dandekar and N Rath (1971)

- First systematic assessment of poverty in India, based on National Sample Survey (NSS) data.
- The previous estimation has stressed subsistence living as a criterion of the poverty line.
- They suggested that the poverty line's criteria must be based on expenditure that would **provide 2250 Calories per day in both rural and urban areas.**
- Rural areas ₹ 180 percapita per annum; Urban areas ₹ 270 per capita per annum

2. Alagh Committee (1979)

- Task Force on "Projections of Minimum Needs and Effective Consumption Demand"
- Poverty line was defined as the per capita consumption expenditure level to meet average per capita daily calorie requirement of **2400 Calories per capita per day in rural areas and 2100 Calories per capita per day in urban areas**
- Based on 1973-74 prices, the Task Force set the rural and urban poverty lines at **49.09 and Rs.56.64 per capita per month at 1973-74 prices.**

3. Lakdawala Committee (1993)

- It did not redefine the poverty line and **retained the separate rural and urban poverty lines** recommended by the Alagh Committee at the national level based on minimum nutritional requirements.
- However, it disaggregated them into **state-specific poverty lines** in order to reflect the inter-state price differentials

4. Tendulkar Committee (2009)

- Shift away from basing the poverty **lines from calorie norms towards target nutritional outcomes instead.**
- Instead of two separate poverty line baskets (PLBs) for rural and urban poverty lines, it recommended **a uniform all-India urban PLB (after adjusting price differentials)** across rural and urban India.
- It recommended using **Mixed Reference Period (MRP)** based estimates, as opposed to Uniform Reference Period (URP) based estimates used in earlier methods for estimating poverty.
- It recommended **incorporation of private expenditure on health and education** while estimating poverty.
- Instead of monthly household consumption, consumption expenditure was broken up into **per person per day consumption**, resulting in the figure of **Rs 32 and Rs 26 a day for urban and rural areas.**

Uniform Recall Period (URP)

- In URP, households are asked to **recall their consumption expenditure over a fixed period of time, usually 30 days.**
- The questionnaire includes a list of food items, non-food items, and services commonly consumed by households in the area.
- The households are asked to report the quantity and price of each item they consumed during the recall period.

Mixed Recall Period (MRP)

- MRP is a method of estimating poverty line that **combines information from a long and short recall period.**
- In MRP, households are asked to **recall their consumption expenditure over a long period, usually 365 days, as well as a short period, usually 30 days.**
- The long recall period captures the seasonal variations in consumption patterns, while the short recall period captures the day-to-day variations.

5. Rangarajan Committee (2012)

- Due to widespread **criticism of Tendulkar Committee approach** as well as due to changing times and aspirations of people of India, Rangarajan Committee was set up in 2012
- It reverted to the practice of having **separate all-India rural and urban poverty line baskets** and deriving state-level rural and urban estimates from these.
- It recommended **separate consumption baskets for rural and urban areas** which include food items that ensure recommended calorie, protein & fat intake and non-food items like clothing, education, health, housing and transport.
- This committee raised the daily per capita expenditure **to Rs 47 for urban and Rs 32 for rural** from Rs 32 and Rs 26 respectively at 2011-12 prices
- Monthly per capita consumption expenditure **of Rs. 972 in rural areas and Rs. 1407 in urban areas** is recommended as the poverty line at the all India level

However, the government **did not take a call on the report** of the Rangarajan Committee.

Vicious cycle of poverty

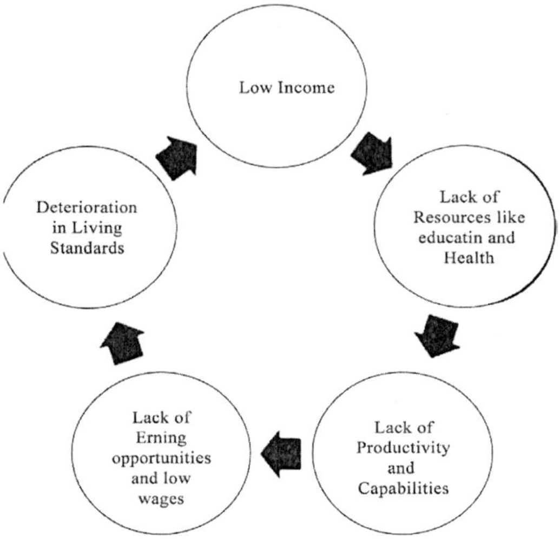

Public Distribution System (PDS)

History

- "World war – II" – war time rationing measure
- 1970s - PDS had evolved into a universal scheme for the distribution of subsidised food
- Till1992 - PDS was a general entitlement scheme for all consumers without any specific target.
- 1992 - Revamped Public Distribution System (RPDS) - to improve its reach in the far-flung, hilly, remote and inaccessible areas where a substantial section of the underprivileged classes lives.
- 1997 - Targeted Public Distribution System (TPDS) with a focus on the poor. (Beneficiaries were divided into BPL & APL)
- 2000 - Antyodaya Anna Yojana (AAY) (Poorest of poor).
- 2013 – NFSA: shift from "welfare based approach" to "right based approach"

Strength of PDS

- Redistribution of grains by **supplying food from surplus regions of the country to deficient regions.**
- Ensures Food Security of the nation by making the **food affordable, accessible and available to the the poor.**

- Provide essential consumer goods at cheap and subsidised prices to the consumers so as **to insulate them from the impact of rising prices / inflation of these commodities.**
- PDS has also been used in India for the distribution of **edible oils, sugar, coal, kerosene and cloth.**
- Ensure **social justice** in the distribution of basic necessities of life.
- The program contributes to reducing poverty levels in India. It ensures that **no one dies from hunger.**
- Special focus towards **poorest of the poor** (Antyodaya Anna Yojana) sections were given additional benefits (35 Kg food grains)

Weakness of PDS – Already discussed in previous class

Recent initiatives in relation to PDS

Direct Benefit Transfer (DBT)

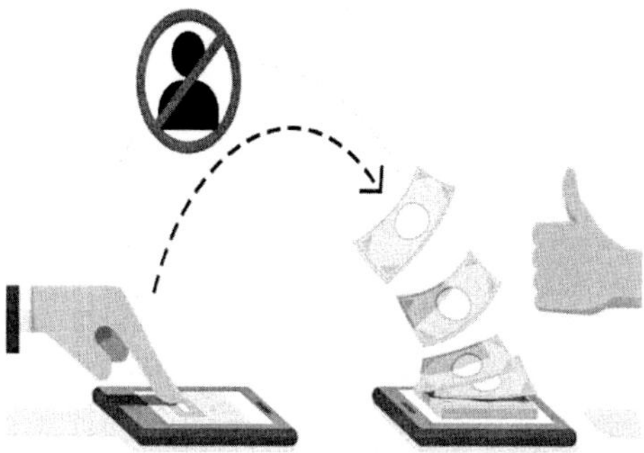

- Reduce the need for huge physical movement of foodgrains
- Provide greater **autonomy to beneficiaries to choose their consumption basket**
- Enhance dietary diversity
- Reduce leakages

Aadhaar Seeding & PDS

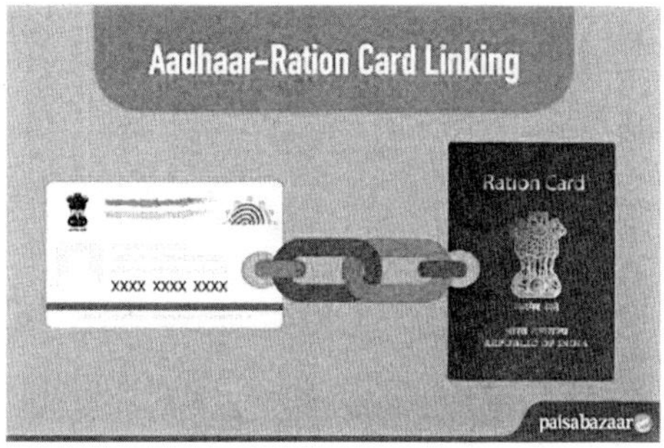

- Welfare programs, where **beneficiaries need to be confirmed before service delivery,** also stand to benefit from UIDAI's verification service.
- Examples of such usages include subsidized food and kerosene delivery to Public Distribution System (PDS) beneficiaries.
- This usage would ensure that **services are delivered to the right beneficiaries only.**

One Nation One Ration Card Scheme

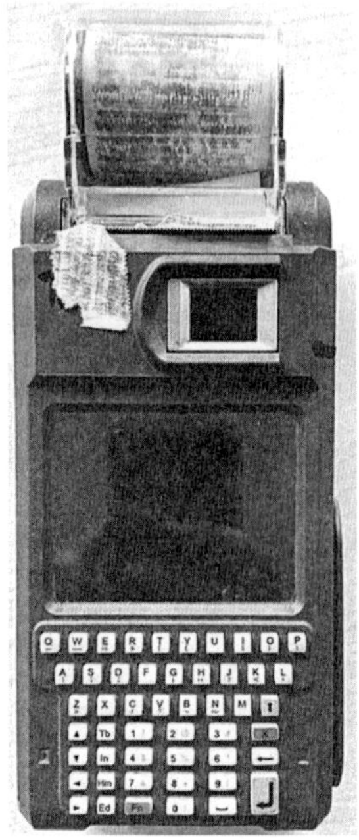

- The scheme which will **allow portability of food security benefits.**
- This means poor migrant workers will be **able to buy subsidized rice and wheat from any ration shop in the country.**
- This scheme will ensure that no poor person is deprived of subsidised grains
- The new system, based on a technological solution, will identify a beneficiary through biometric authentication on **electronic Point of Sale (ePoS) devices installed at the FPSs,** and enable that person to purchase the quantity of foodgrains to which she is entitled under the NFSA.
- **Annavitran portal** enables a migrant worker or his family to avail the benefits of PDS outside their district but within their state.

8

Relation of Food Production to National Dietary Guidelines and Food Consumption Pattern

Previous Year Questions

1. *What are the different 'National Dietary Guidelines' of India? What is your opinion on balanced diet of Indians? (20M, CSE 2021)*
2. *Classify foods on the basis of their function. Write down a balanced diet for a sedentary man & woman in India (10M, CS 2023)*

National Dietary Guidelines

Recommended dietary allowance (RDA) is defined as ***"the nutrient present in the diet which satisfies the daily requirement of nearly all individuals in a population".***

What is a Balanced Diet?

- A balanced diet is one which provides all the nutrients in required amounts and proper proportions.
- The quantities of foods needed to meet the nutrient requirements vary with age, gender, physiological status and physical activity.

A Balanced Diet Should Provide Around

- 50-60% of total calories from carbohydrates, preferably from complex carbohydrates,
- about 10-15% from proteins and
- 20-30% from both visible and invisible fat.

National Dietary Guidelines of India

1. **Eat variety of foods** to ensure a balanced diet.
2. Ensure provision of extra food and healthcare to **pregnant and lactating women.**
3. Promote **exclusive breastfeeding** for six months and encourage breastfeeding till two years or as long as one can.

4. Feed home based **semi solid foods to the infant after six months.**
5. Ensure adequate and **appropriate diets for children and adolescents,** both in health and sickness.
6. Eat plenty of **vegetables and fruits.**
7. Ensure moderate use of **edible oils and animal foods** and very less use of **ghee/ butter/ vanaspati.**
8. **Avoid overeating** to prevent overweight and obesity.
9. **Exercise regularly and be physically active** to maintain ideal body weight.
10. **Restrict salt** intake to minimum.
11. Ensure the use of **safe and clean foods.**
12. Adopt right **pre-cooking processes and appropriate cooking methods.**
13. **Drink plenty of water** and take beverages in moderation.
14. **Minimize the use of processed foods** rich in salt, sugar and fats.
15. Include **micronutrient-rich foods in the diets of elderly people** to enable them to be fit and active.

What is Sedentary Lifestyle?

- A lifestyle type, in which one is **physically inactive and does little or no physical movement and or exercise.**
- Sedentary behavior is defined as any waking behavior such as sitting or leaning with an **energy expenditure of 1.5 metabolic equivalent task (MET) or less**
- When someone **spends six or more hours per day** sitting or lying down

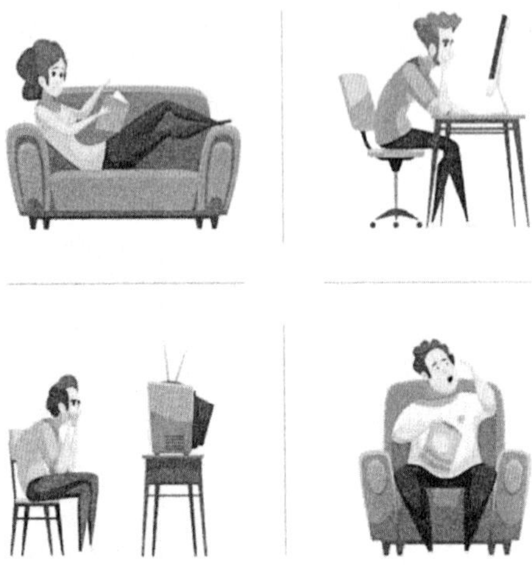

- **Examples :** Television viewing, playing video games, using a computer, sitting at school or work, and sitting while commuting

Balanced Diet for a Sedentary Man & Woman in India

1. Action plan for a Balanced Diet

- The most important rule for healthy eating is **not to skip any meal.**

- Skipping meals lowers your metabolic rate. Especially, **never skip breakfast.**
- **Limit the number of times** you eat out.
- **Limit stimulants** such as caffeine and alcohol.
- Intake **raw foods such as salads, fruits and vegetable juices**

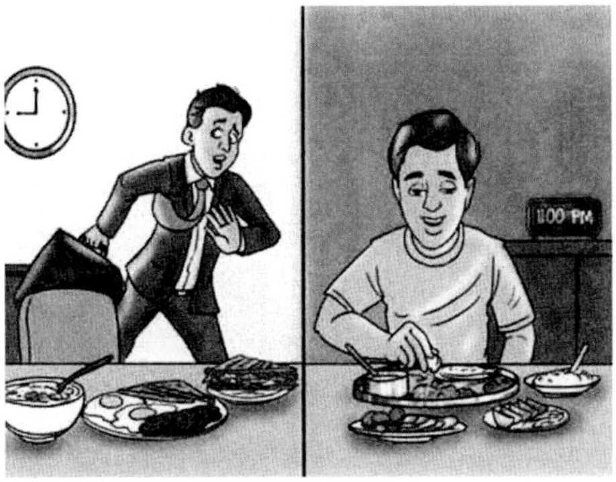

- **Avoid fried foods** or take off the extra oil.
- Choose **reduced-fat ingredients** such as low-fat cheese or salad dressing.
- Drink lots of water.

2. Add fresh fruits and vegetables to your diet

- Include fruits such as **bananas, apples with hot or cold breakfast cereals**
- **Snack with fruit** rather than sweets, biscuits, cookies etc
- Snack on **cherry tomatoes, carrot and cucumber sticks, dried apricots or nuts**

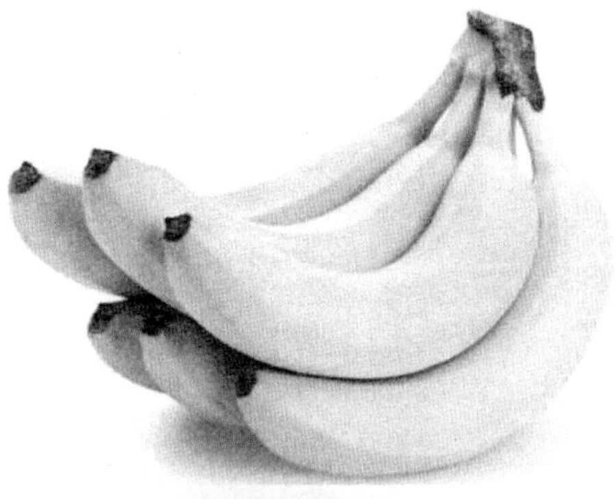

3. Eat the right carbohydrates

- Most people think that all starchy foods are fattening.
- But starchy foods contain a lot of fiber giving you that full, satisfied feeling.
- Eat **brown rice, whole-grain pasta, sweet potatoes or wholegrain bread** whenever possible.

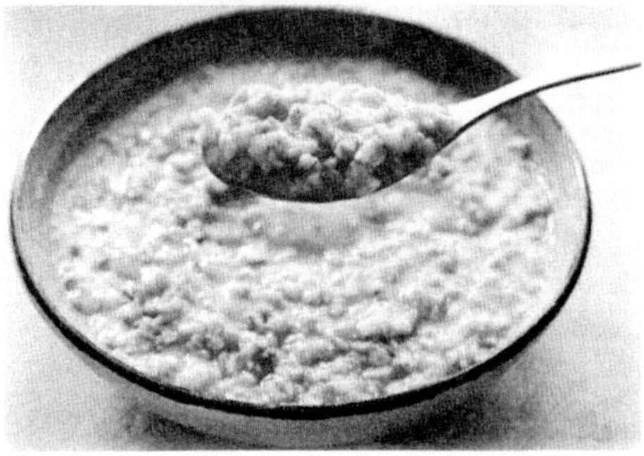

- If you have cereals for breakfast, **choose porridge or oatmeal without sugar.**

4. Cut down on sugary foods

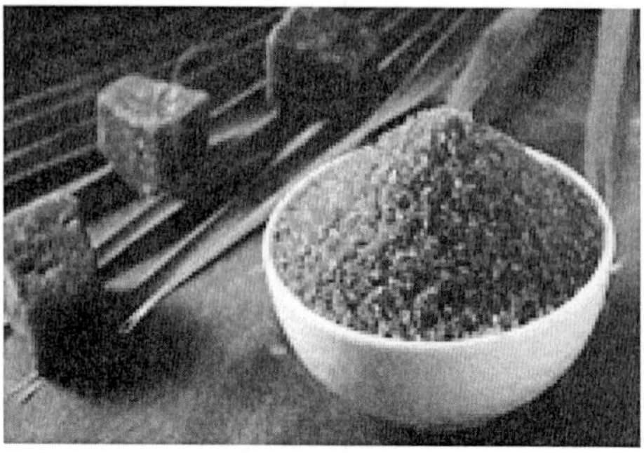

- Replace **sugary drinks with water**
- Avoid using **sugar in coffee, tea or breakfast cereals**
- If you have to sweeten, try **natural sugar alternative (Jaggery).**

5. Cut down on Fatty foods

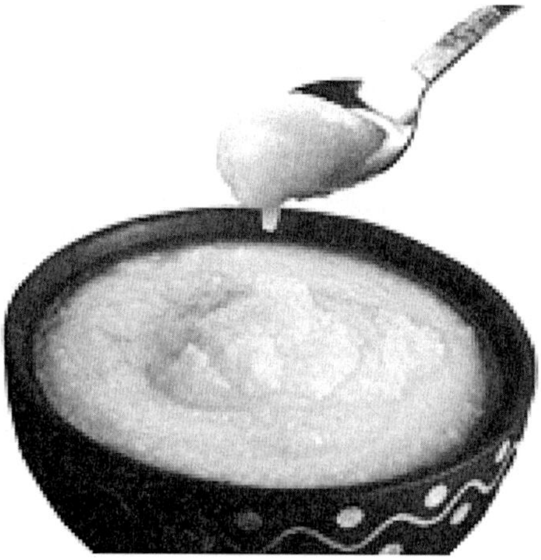

- A diet which is too rich in fat can **increase the risk of heart disease and stroke.**
- **Avoid saturated fats** like butter, ghee and/or margarine
- **Grill, bake, poach or boil food** instead of frying
- If you fry food, **use unsaturated oil** and remove excess oil before eating
- Be aware of hidden fat in **pastries, chocolate, cakes and biscuits.**
- Choose **low-fat milk, cheeses and yogurts** over full-fat varieties

6. Eat the right type of Protein

- Eat fish rich in Omega-3 fatty acids, like salmon and mackerel at least once a week or more.
- Add beans and Soy products to your diet for a low-fat source of protein, fiber, vitamins & minerals

Sample Meal Plan for Adult Men Sedentary

Meal Time	Food group	Row	Cooked Recipe	Servings Amounts
Breakfast	Milk	100 ml	Milk	1/2 Cup
	Sugar	15g	Tea or Coffee	2 Cups 1 Cup
	Cereals	70 g	Breakfast item	
	Pulses	20 g		
Lunch	Cereals	120 g	Rice	2 Cups
			Pulkas	2 Nos.
	Pulses	20 g	Dhal	1/2 Cup
	Vegetables	150g	Veg. curry	3/4 Cup
	Vegetables	50 g	Veg. salad	7-8 Slices
	Milk	100 ml	Curd	1/2 Cup
Tea	Cereals			
	Milk	50 ml	Tea	1 Cup
	Sugar			
Dinner	Cereals	120 g	Rice	2 Cups
			Pulkas	2 Nos.
	Pulses	20 g	Dhal	1/2 Cup
	Vegetables	150 g	Veg. curry	3/4 Cup
	Milk (Curd)	50 ml		
	Vegetables	50 g		
	Fruit	100 g	Seasonal	1 Medium

1 Cup = 200 ml

Note: For Non-Vegetarians - Substitute one pulse portion with one portion of egg/ meat/chicken/fish

Use 25 g visible fat and <5g salt during preparation of meal per day.

Breakfast Items: Idlli - 4 Nos./ Dosa - 3 Nos./ Upma - 1-1/2 Cup / Bread - 4 Slices/ Porridge -2 Cups/ Corn flakes with milk - 2 Cups.

Snacks: Poha - 1 Cup/Toast -2 Slices Dhokla- 4 Nos.

Sample Meal Plan for Adult Women Sedentary

Meal Time	Food group	Row	Cooked Recipe	Servings Amounts
Breakfast	Milk	100 ml	Milk	1/2 Cup
	Sugar	10g	Tea or Coffee	2 Cups 1 Cup
	Cereals	50 g	Breakfast item	
	Pulses	20 g		
Lunch	Cereals	100 g	Rice	1 Cups
			Pulkas	2 Nos.
	Pulses	20 g	Dhal	1/2 Cup
	Vegetables	100g	Veg. curry	1/2 Cup
	Vegetables	50 g	Veg. salad	7-8 Slices
	Milk	100 ml	Curd	1/2 Cup
Tea	Cereals	50g	Snack	
	Milk	50 ml	Tea	1 Cup
	Sugar	10g		
Dinner	Cereals	100 g	Rice	2 Cups
			Phulkas	2 Nos.
	Pulses	20 g	Dhal	1/2 Cup
	Vegetables	100 g	Veg. curry	1/2 Cup
	Milk (Curd)	50 ml		
	Vegetables	50 g		
	Fruit	100 g	Seasonal	1 Medium

1 Cup = 200 ml

Note: For Non-Vegetarians - Substitute one pulse portion with one portion of egg/ meat/chicken/fish

Use 20 g visible fat and <5g salt during preparation of meal per day.

Breakfast Items: Idlli - 3 Nos./ Dosa - 2 Nos./ Upma - 1 Cup / Bread - 3 Slices/ Porridge -1-1/2 Cups/ Corn flakes with milk -1-1/2 Cups.

Snacks: Poha - 1 Cup/Toast -2 Slices Dhokla- 4 Nos.

9

Food Based Dietary Approaches to Eliminate Hunger

Previous Year Questions

1. *Differentiate between protective foods and energy foods. (10M, IFoS-2015)*
2. *What do you mean by 'hunger' and 'hidden hunger'? Comment on various strategies in combating hunger. (15M, CSE 2021)*
3. *Classify foods on the basis of their function (5M, 2023)*

Energy Rich Foods

Energy Rich Foods	**Carbohydrates & Fats**
Whole grajn cereals, millets	Protein, fibre, minerals, calcium, lron B-complex vitamins
Vegetable oils, ghee, butter	Fat soluble vitamins, essential fatty acids
Nuts and oilseeds	Proteins, vitamins, minerals
Sugars	Nil

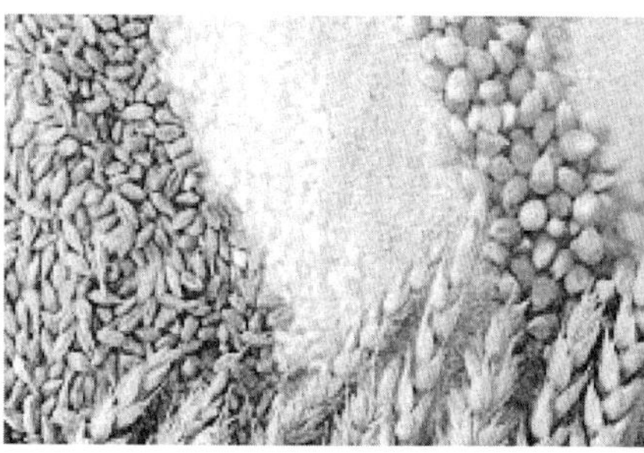

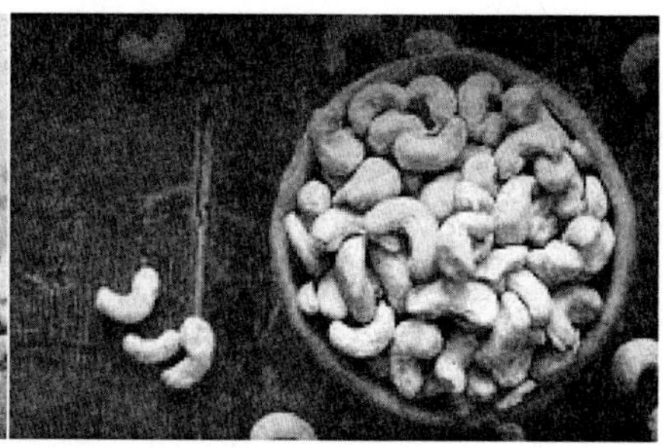

Body building foods

Body Building Foods	**Proteins**
Pulses, nuts and oilseeds	B-complex vitamins, invisible fat, fibre
Milk and Milk products	Calcium, vitamin A. riboflavin, vitamin B12
Meat, fish, poultry	B-complex vitamins, iron, iodine, fat

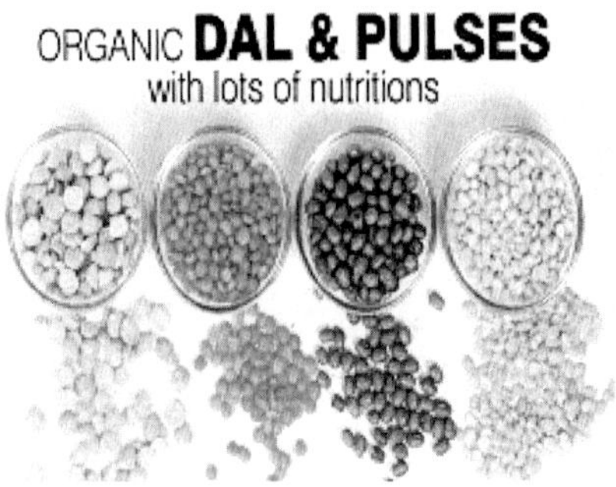

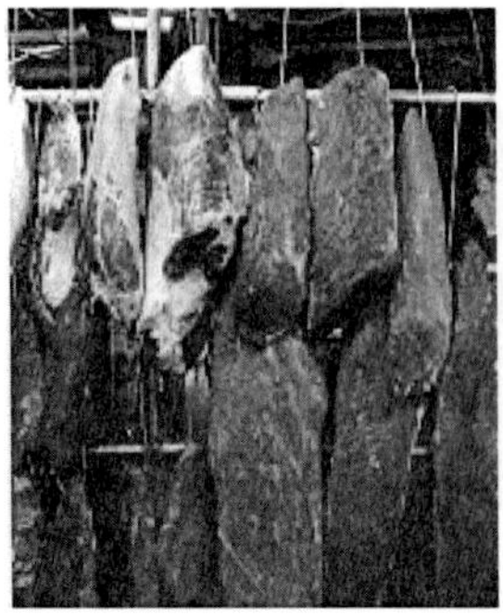

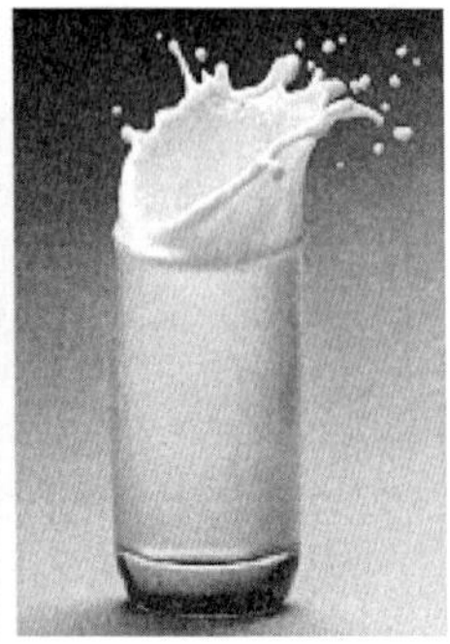

Protective foods

Protective Foods	Vitamins and Minerals
Green leafy vegetables	Antioxidants, fibre and other carotenoids
Other vegetables and fruits	Fibre, sugar and antioxidants
Eggs, milk and milk products and flesh foods	Protein and fat

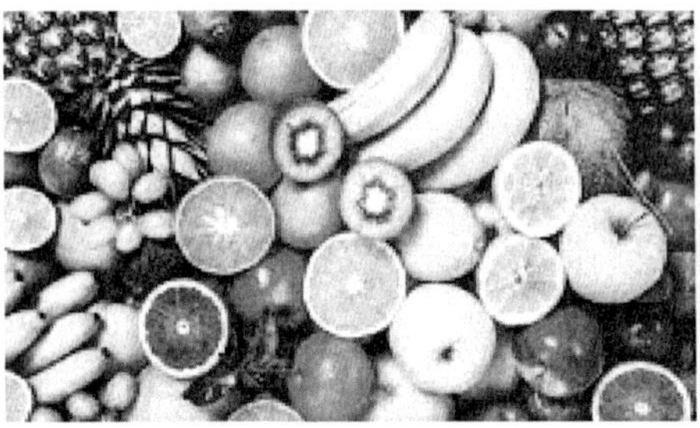

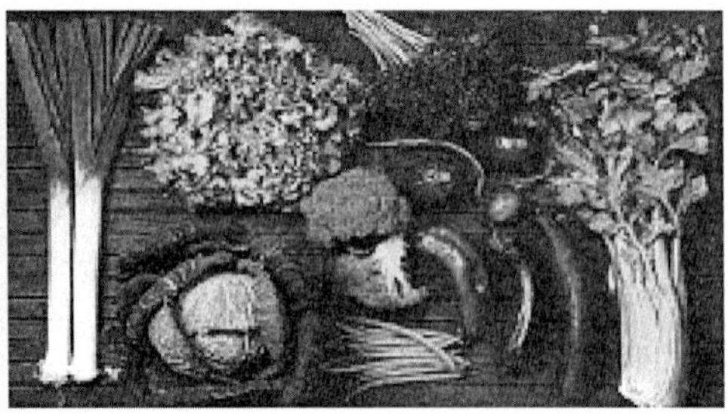

What is Hunger ?

- Hunger is defined as ***"a condition in which a person does not have the physical or financial capability to eat sufficient food to meet basic nutritional needs for a sustained period. In common parlance, hunger refers to discomfort due to a lack of food".***
- India ranked 107 out of 121 countries in **Global hunger index**
- Prevalence of undernourishment has also risen in the country from 14.6% in 2018-2020 to **16.3% in 2019-2021**
- According to NFHS-5 survey, The **zero-food prevalence** was 30% for infants aged 6-11 months, 13% among 12-17 months old, and 8% among 18-23 months old children
- Going without food for an entire day at this critical period of a child's development can have severe implications

Global Hunger Index

- The Global Hunger Index (GHI) is a tool for comprehensively measuring and tracking hunger at global, regional, and national levels.
- GHI scores are based on the values of four component indicators:
  - Undernourishment
  - Child stunting
  - Child wasting
  - Child mortality
- The GHI score is calculated on a 100-point scale reflecting the severity of hunger - **zero is the best score (implies no hunger) and 100 is the worst.**
- The GHI is prepared by European NGOs of **Concern Worldwide and Welthungerhilfe.**
- The GHI is an annual report and each set of GHI scores **uses data from a 5-year period.** The 2022 GHI scores are calculated using data from 2017 to 2021

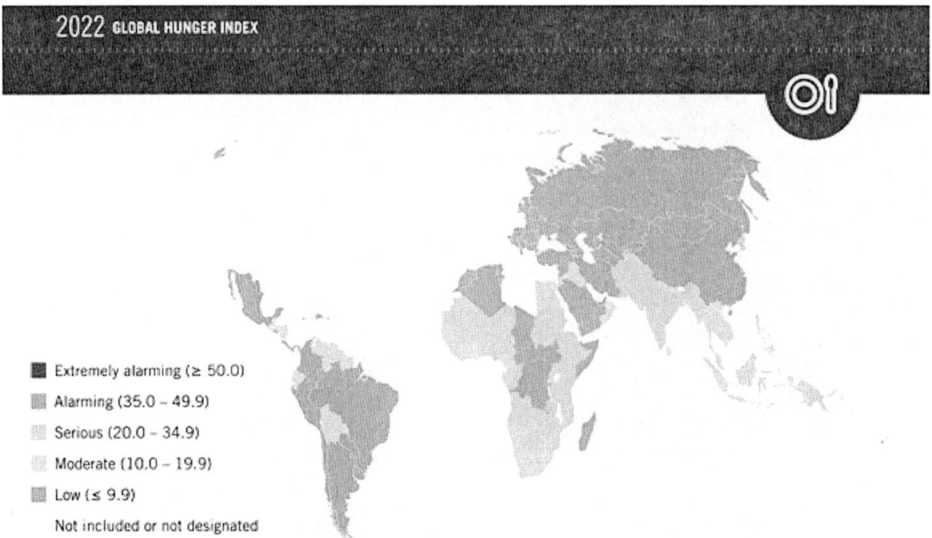
2022 GLOBAL HUNGER INDEX
Extremely alarming (≥ 50.0)
Alarming (35.0 – 49.9)
Serious (20.0 – 34.9)
Moderate (10.0 – 19.9)
Low (≤ 9.9)
Not included or not designated

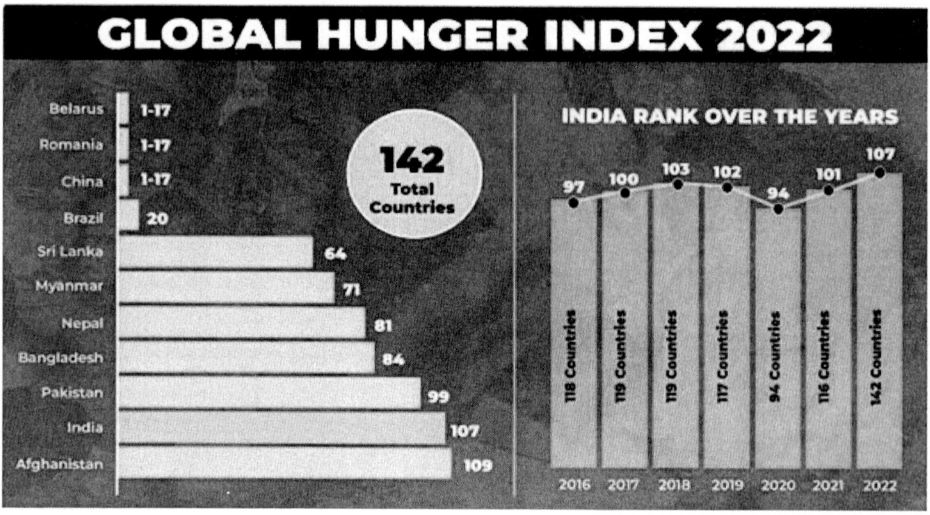
GLOBAL HUNGER INDEX 2022
Belarus 1-17
Romania 1-17
China 1-17
Brazil 20
Sri Lanka 64
Myanmar 71
Nepal 81
Bangladesh 84
Pakistan 99
India 107
Afghanistan 109
142 Total Countries
INDIA RANK OVER THE YEARS
97 100 103 102 94 101 107
118 Countries
119 Countries
119 Countries
117 Countries
94 Countries
116 Countries
142 Countries
2016 2017 2018 2019 2020 2021 2022

Hidden Hunger

- Hidden hunger is a form of undernutrition that occurs when intake and absorption of **vitamins and minerals (such as zinc, iodine, and iron) are too low** to sustain good health and development (IFPRI).
- The 'hidden hunger' due to micronutrient deficiency does not produce hunger as we know it. You might not feel it in the belly, but it strikes at the core of your health and vitality.

Hidden Hunger in India (as Per Global Hunger Report)	
Iodine deficiency	25%
Anemia among pregnant women	54%
Anemia among children under 5	59%
Vit.A deficiency	62%

Clinical Signs

- While clinical signs of hidden hunger, such as **night blindness due to vitamin A deficiency and goiter from inadequate iodine intake,** become visible once deficiencies become severe, the health and development of a much larger share of the population is affected by **less obvious "invisible" effects.**
- That is why micronutrient deficiencies are often referred to as hidden hunger.

Factors Responsible for it

- Poor diet,
- Increased micronutrient needs during certain life stages, such as pregnancy and lactation,
- Health problems such as diseases, infections, or parasites.

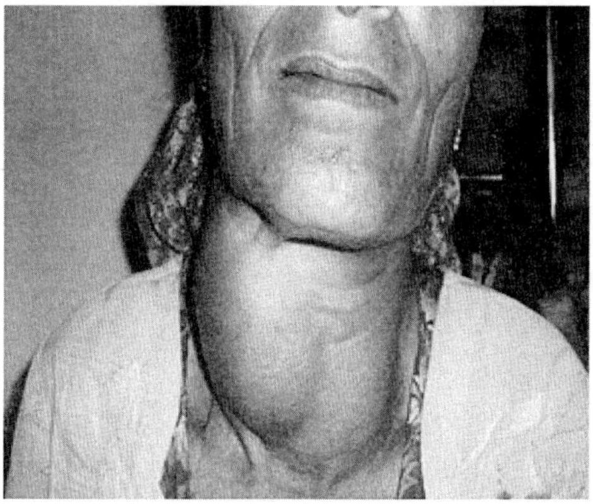

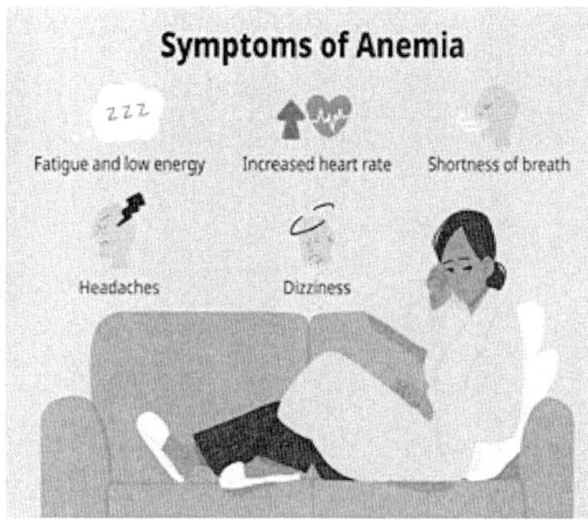

10

Nutrient Deficiency (a) Micro Nutrient Deficiency, Protein Energy Malnutrition or Protein Calorie Malnutrition (PEM or PCM), (b) Micro Nutrient Deficiency and HRD in Context of Work Capacity of Women and Children

Previous Year Questions

1. *Discuss the iron and protein malnutrition in India. Describe the dietary pattern for mitigating the above-said malnutrition. (15M, IFoS-2022)*
2. *What is protein energy malnutrition? Give micronutrient deficiency in women and children. (20M, CSE 2017)*
3. *How are vitamins classified? Name the blood clotting vitamin. Give its various functions and sources. (10M, 150W, CSE 2019)*
4. *What do you mean by nutrient deficiency? Explain the micro-nutrient deficiency in context of work capacity of women and children. (12.5M, CSE 2015)*

Protein Energy Malnutrition

- As per the World Health Organization, protein energy malnutrition is a **"disparity between the supply of protein and energy and the body's need for them to guarantee healthy development/ optimal growth"**
- It affects **children under 5 mostly belonging to the poor** underprivileged communities.
- PEM is particularly serious during the **post-weaning stage** and is often associated with infection.

- The term PEM covers a wide spectrum of clinical stages ranging from the **severe forms like kwashiorkor and marasmus to the milder forms** in which the main detectable manifestation is growth retardation.

Feature	**Kwashiorkor**	**Marasmus**
Deficiency	Protein	Energy
Appearance	Sugar Baby	Very Thin
Growth	Retarded	Retarded
Edema	Pitting Edema Present	Absent
Activity	Apathetic, Less Active and Refuse to eat	Notably Apathetic, Less Active and Interested
Appetite	Poor	Good
Muscle Wasting	Present	Markedly Present
Mental Changes	Common	Uncommon
Hepatomegaly	Present	Absent
Infections	More prone	Less prone
Hair Changes	Common, Sparse and Scanty	Uncommon
Anemia	Moderate-Severe	Mild generally
Subcutaneous fat	Reduced	Absent
Face	Moon-shaped	Monkey-facies

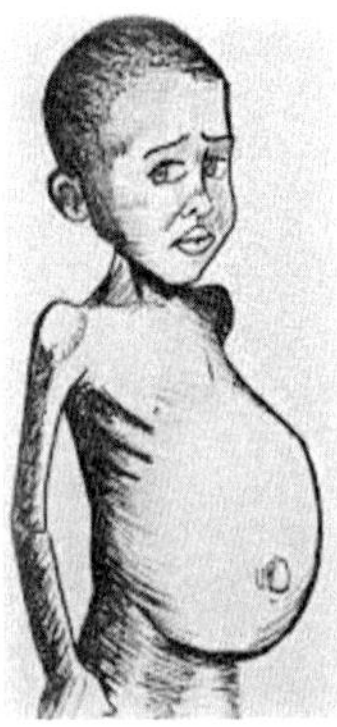

Kwashiorkor

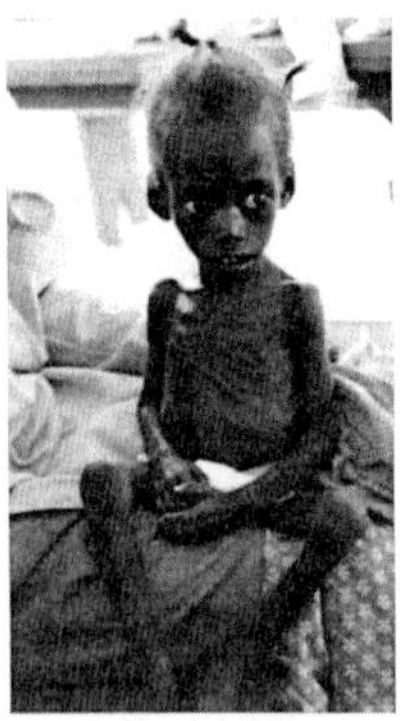

Marasmus

Micronutrients

- Micronutrients are nutrients (vitamins and minerals) needed by the body in **very small amounts.**
- However, their **impact on a body's health are critical**, and deficiency in any of them can cause severe and even life-threatening conditions.
- They perform a range of functions, including enabling the body **to produce enzymes, hormones and other substances needed** for normal growth and development.

- Deficiencies in **iron, vitamin A and iodine** are the most common around the world, particularly in children and pregnant women.
- **Low- and middle-income counties** bear the disproportionate burden of micronutrient deficiencies.

Vitamins

Vitamins are chemical compounds that are required in small amounts with our regular diet

Classification

1. Fat-Soluble Vitamins

- Vitamin A, D, E and K are fat-soluble.
- These are stored in adipose tissues and hence are called fat-soluble vitamins.

2. Water-Soluble Vitamins

- Vitamins in B-group and vitamin C are water-soluble and cannot be stored in our bodies as they pass with the water in urine.
- These vitamins must be supplied to our bodies with regular diets.

Functions of Vitamins

Vitamin A – Hardening of the cornea in the eye, night blindness.

Vitamin B1 – Deficiency may cause beriberi and dwarfism.

Vitamin B2 – Deficiency can cause disorders in the digestive system, skin burning sensations, and cheilosis.

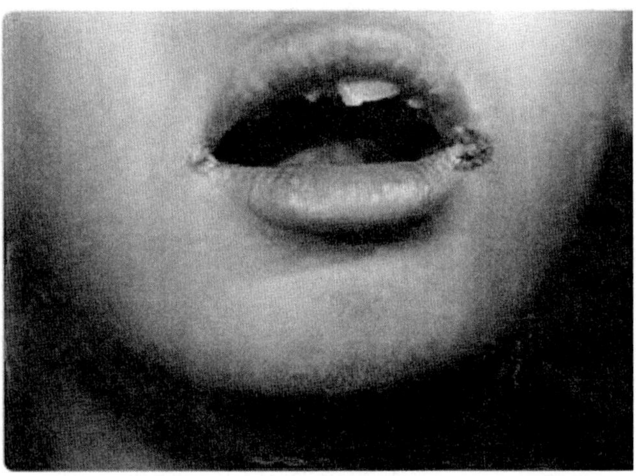

Vitamin B6 – Deficiency of B6 causes convulsions, conjunctivitis, and sometimes neurological disorders.

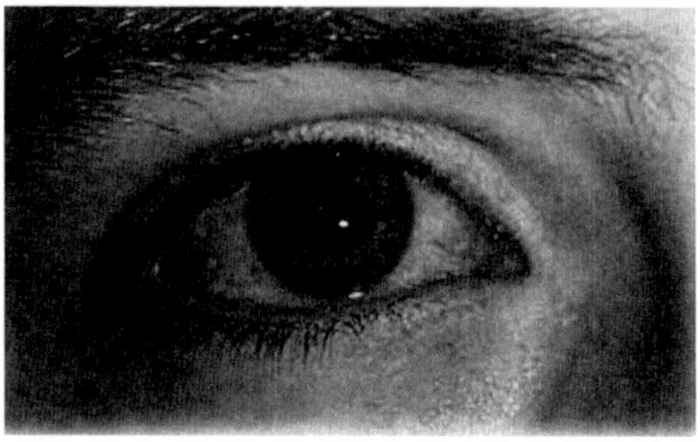

Vitamin B12 – Its deficiency can cause pernicious anaemia and a decrease in red blood cells in haemoglobin.

Vitamin C – It is a water-soluble vitamin, its deficiency causes bleeding in gums and scurvy.

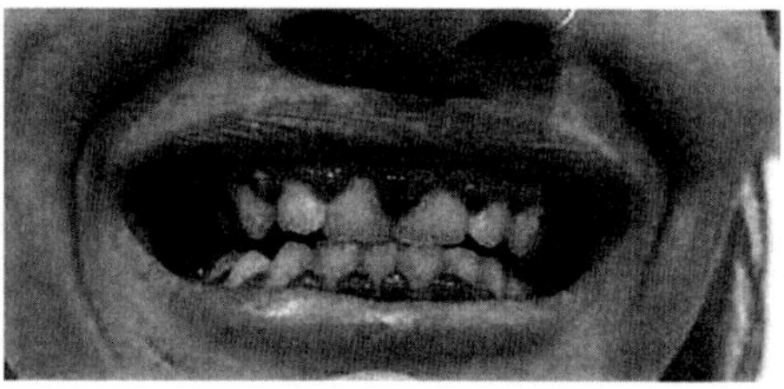

Vitamin D – It is obtained by our body when exposed to sunlight. Its deficiency causes improper growth of bones, soft bones in kids, and rickets.

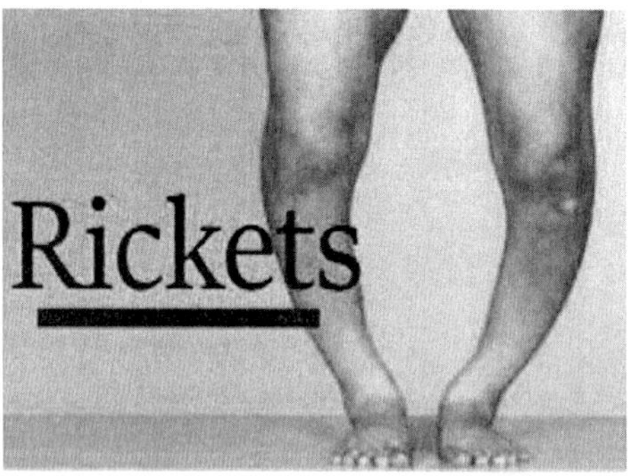

Vitamin E – Deficiency of vitamin E leads to weakness in muscles and increases the fragility of red blood cells.

Vitamin K – It plays an important role in blood clotting. The deficiency of vitamin K increases the time taken by the blood to clot. Severe deficiency may cause death due to excessive blood loss in case of a cut or an injury.

Name	Solubility	Food Sources	Deficiency Diseaes
Vitamin A	Fat	Green leafy vegetables, ripe yellow fruits, guava, milk, liver, nuts, tomatoes, oranges, carrots, broccoli, watermelon etc.	Hyperkeratosis, night blindness, and keratomalacia
Vitamin Bl (Thiamine)	Water	Fresh fruits, potatoes, sweet potatoes, peas, corn, cashew nuts, wheat, milk, black beans, dates etc.	Beriberi
Vitamin B2 (Riboflavin)	Water	Banana, dates, mushrooms, grapes, mangoes, peas, pumpkin, popcorn etc.	Slow growth, sore eye
Vitamin B3 (Niacin)	Water	Meat, fish, eggs, milk products, cereals, mushroom, guava etc.	Pellagra
Vitamin C	Water	Fresh fruits, black currant, broccoli, goat milk and chestnuts.	Scurvy
Vitamin D	Fat	Fish, egg, liver, beef, cod, chicken breast etc.	Rickets and Osteomalacia
Vitamin E	Fat	Potatoes, pumpkin, guava, mango, milk, nuts, seeds etc.	Heart problems, Haemolysis and sterility
Vitamin K	Fat	Tomatoes, broccoli, chestnuts, cashew nuts, beef, lamb, mangoes, grapes etc.	Haemorrhage

Prevalence of Anaemia

- Iron deficiency anemia is due to **insufficient iron.**
- Without enough iron, your body can't produce enough of a substance in **red blood cells that enables them to carry oxygen** (hemoglobin).
- As a result, iron deficiency anemia may leave you tired and short of breath.

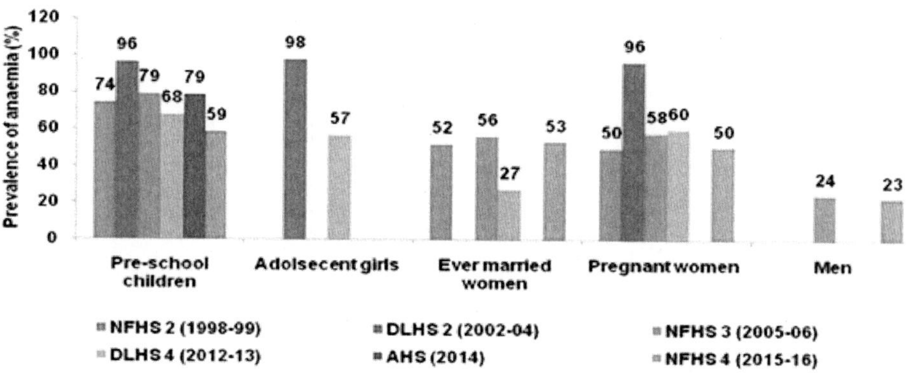

- The prevalence of anaemia among six groups as per the National Family Health Survey 5 (2019-21):
- 25.0% in men (15-49 years) and 57.0% in women (15-49 years),
- 31.1% in adolescent boys (15-19 yrs), 59.1% in adolescent girls,
- **52.2% in pregnant women (15-49 years) and 67.1% in children (6-59 months).**

Govt. initiative - Weekly Iron Folic Acid Supplementation (WIFS)

- The Programme is being implemented to meet the challenge of **high prevalence and incidence of anaemia amongst adolescent girls and boys.**
- The intervention under WIFS includes **supervised weekly ingestion of Iron Folic Acid (IFA) tablet.**

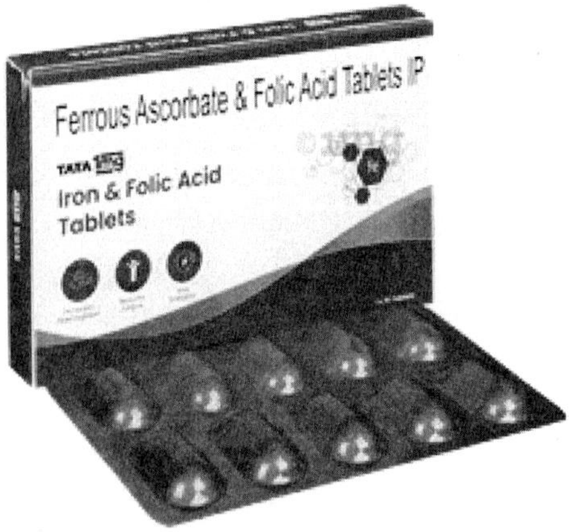

11

Food Grain Productivity and Food Security

Previous Year Questions

1. *What is food security? Why is it essential? Describe the current food security system in India. (10M, CSE 2022)*
2. *What is food security? Indicate the major constraints in food procurement and distribution. (10M, CSE 2017)*

Difference Between Production and Productivity

- Production is **total quantity produced** in an area.
- Productivity is the **quantity produced in one unit area.**
- For example, total area is 10 hectares and the quantity produced is 15000 kg.
- Here, the production is 15000kg.
- Productivity is 1500 Kg per hectare.

Table 1. Productivity of Food-grains in India (1990-91 to 2019-20)(In kg/ hectare)

Year	Rice	Wheat	Coarse Cereals	Total Cereals	Pulses	Total food grain
1990-91	1740	2281	900	1571	578	1380
1991-92	1751	2394	778	1574	533	1382
1992-93	1744	2327	1063	1654	573	1457
1993-94	1888	2380	939	1701	598	1501
1994-95	1911	2559	929	1763	610	1546
1995-96	1797	2483	940	1703	552	1491
1996-97	1882	2679	1072	1831	635	1614
1997-98	1900	2485	986	1775	567	1552
1998-99	1921	2590	1068	1856	634	1627
1999-00	1986	2778	1034	1925	635	1704
2000-01	1901	2708	1027	1844	544	1626
2001-02	2079	2762	1131	1980	607	1734

2002-03	1744	2610	966	1753	543	1535
2003-04	2077	2713	1221	1983	635	1727
2004-05	1984	2602	1153	1903	577	1652
2005-06	2102	2619	1172	1968	598	1715
2006-07	2131	2708	1182	2021	612	1756
2007-08	2202	2802	1431	2151	625	1860
2008-09	2178	2907	1459	2183	659	1909
2009-10	2125	2839	1212	2075	630	1798
2010-11	2239	2988	1531	2256	691	1930
2011-12	2393	3177	1590	2415	699	2078
2012-13	2461	3117	1617	2449	789	2129
2013-14	2424	3075	1677	2438	764	2101
2014-15	2390	2872	1729	2373	744	2070
2015-16	2400	3034	1579	2392	656	2056
2016-17	2494	3200	1750	2525	786	2129
2017-18	2576	3368	1934	2657	853	2235
2018-19	2638	3533	1944	2752	757	2286
2019-20	2705	3421	1976	2756	817	2325

Food Security

- Based on the 1996 World Food Summit, Food security is defined as "when all people, at all times, have physical and economic access to sufficient safe and nutritious food that meets their dietary needs and food preferences for an active and healthy life".

It has the Following Dimensions:

1. **Availability:** It means food production within the country, food imports and the stock stored in government granaries.
2. **Accessibility:** It means food is within reach of every person without any discrimination.
3. **Affordability:** It implies that having enough money to buy sufficient, safe and nutritious food to meet one's dietary needs.

Why Food Security is Essential ?

- Food security concerns can be traced back to **the famine experience that Bengal had undergone in 1943** during the British rule in India.
- During this famine, around **2 to 3 million people perished due to starvation**. Food security is essential in a country to make sure that food is available to all anytime and also to do away with the problem of starvation.

- Food security is very essential, especially for those people living **below the poverty line** to assure them that they have access to food in times of danger and that not only the privileged people have access to food items.
- Food security is also essential so that during times of natural calamities such as **drought, earthquakes, famine, etc** when the production of food grain decreases and the leftover stock prices increase, people can be supplied with food.
- During this **shortage of food, when food prices go up**, problems of starvation may occur among the people when such a situation stretches over a long period of time.

Food Security System in India

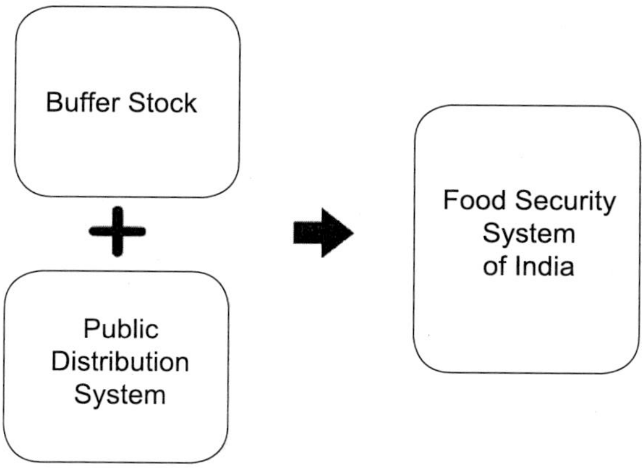

Buffer Stock

- The concept of buffer stock was first introduced during the **4th Five Year Plan** (1969-74)
- Earlier this concept was termed as "**Buffer Norms and Strategic Reserve**".
- At present, the Government of India prefers to use the term – **Food grain stocking norms** –***the level of stock in the Central Pool that is sufficient to meet the operational requirement of food grains and exigencies at any point of time.***

Buffer Norms w.e.f. 01.07.2017

(Figure in lakh MT)

As on	Operational Stock			Strategic Reserve		Grand
	Rice	Wheat	Total	Rice	Wheat	Total
1st April	**115.80**	**44.60**	**160.40**	20.00	30.00	210.40
1st July	115.40	245.80	361.20	20.00	30.00	411.20
1st October	82.5O	175.20	257.70	20.00	30.00	307.70
1st January	56.10	108.00	164.10	20.00	30.00	214.10

Objectives of Buffer Stock

- For monthly release of food grains for supply through **Targeted Public Distribution System (TPDS) and Other Welfare Schemes (OWS)**
- For meeting emergency situations arising out of **unexpected crop failure, natural disasters, etc.**
- For the purpose of **Price stabilisation or market intervention** to augment supply, so as to help moderate the open market prices.
- The crops are procured at MSP so that the **farmers do not suffer negatively** for producing more.
- In times of deficit, government releases the buffer stocks in a phased manner so that interests of the **consumers do not suffer**.

Who Decides the Buffer Stock in India

- **The Cabinet Committee on Economic Affairs** fixes the minimum buffer norms on quarterly basis: i.e. as on every financial year
  - 1st April,
  - 1st July,
  - 1st October and
  - 1st January
- Presently, stocking norms fixed by Government of India on 22.01.2015 comprise of:

1. **Operational stocks:** Meeting monthly distributional requirement under TPDS & OWS
2. **Food security stocks/reserves:** for meeting shortfall in procurement.

How the Public Distribution System Works

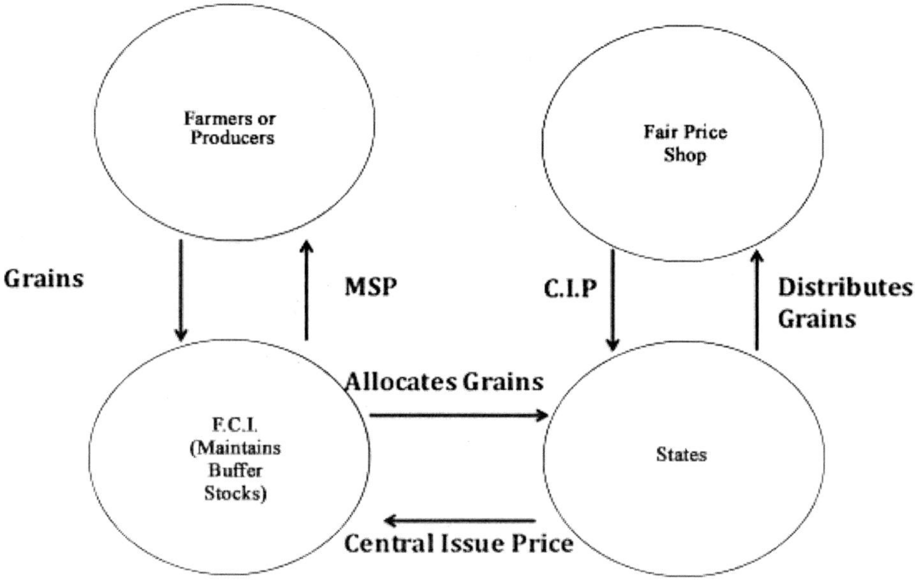

Bibliography

Official website of Ministry of Agriculture & Farmers' Welfare (https://agriwelfare.gov.in)
Official website of Ministry of Women and Child Development (https://wcd.nic.in)
Official website of Ministry of Consumer Affairs, Food and Public Distribution (https://dfpd.gov.in)